OUTLIVING
Heart Disease

OUTLIVING
Heart Disease

The

10 New Rules

for

Prevention and Treatment

Richard A. Stein, MD

Professor of Medicine and Director of the
Urban Community Cardiology Program,
New York University School of Medicine, New York City

Newmarket Press • New York

Updated paperback edition 2008

This book is published in the United States of America.

ISBN: 978-1-55704-788-5

10 9 8 7 6 5 4 3 2 1

Library of Congress Cataloging-in-Publication Data

Stein, Richard A., MD
  Outliving heart disease : the 10 new rules for prevention and treatment / Richard A. Stein.—1st ed.
      p. cm.
  Includes index.
  ISBN 1-55704-594-1 (cloth : alk. paper)
  1. Heart—Diseases—Prevention—Popular works. 2. Heart—Diseases—Treatment—Popular works. I. Title.
  RC672.S72 2005
  616.1'205—dc22

QUANTITY PURCHASES

Companies, professional groups, clubs, and other organizations may qualify for special terms when ordering quantities of this title. For information or a catalog, write Special Sales Department, Newmarket Press, 18 East 48th Street, New York, NY 10017; call (212) 832-3575; fax (212) 832-3629; or e-mail info@newmarketpress.com.

www.newmarketpress.com

Designed by Betty Lew

Manufactured in the United States of America.

This book is dedicated to my wife, Roselle Shubin.
Her love of life, her acts of caring, and her passionate
sense of fairness are attributes I continually try to emulate.
The love that we share is a precious gift,
for which I am thankful every day.

Our children, Ken and Beth, Beth's husband, Chris,
and our grandson, Charlie, are a truly amazing source
of pride, delight, and energy.
My mom, Jean, whom I remember every day, and
my dad, Jacob, have given us the most precious gifts
parents could give—love, self-esteem, and
their avid interest in our lives.
Roselle's parents, Jeanette and Joe,
gave us their love, their time and joy,
and by example their profound sense
of goodness to all.

Contents

Preface

OUTLIVING HEART DISEASE

I remember clearly when I first made the decision to become a cardiologist and focus my work on preventing heart attacks. I had just begun my internship at Kings County Hospital in Brooklyn, New York. My wife, Roselle, and I lived a block away from the hospital and we were eating dinner (spaghetti, so that we could save money for a trip to Italy). It was my first night on call and I remember worrying about spilling tomato sauce on my still-stiff white pants and jacket. Like a kid on his first day of school, I was excited but nervous, wondering what the evening would bring. I was twenty-five years old.

At about 8:30 my beeper went off: my first patient had arrived in the ER. By the time I got there he'd been moved to the acute care room. Five residents were gathered around, trying to resuscitate him as he lay face up on the stretcher. He looked like a young man, perhaps in his late thirties. A breathing tube had been placed in his throat and connected to a respirator. Two intravenous lines were running into him and a defibrillator was being used to shock his heart at least three more times while I stood by. An electrocardiogram (EKG) machine was also running, its long paper strip collecting on the floor. One of the residents looked up and saw me, and from his expression I knew that their work was done. They stopped what had been an aggressive and prolonged effort to restore the patient's heartbeat.

Since I arrived before he was pronounced dead, he was technically my first admission. It was my job to tell his wife, who was waiting outside the room, that her husband had died. I had never done that, and I truly do not remember how I told her or what I said. We sat for a while and she told me that her husband, a science teacher at a nearby high school, had been on the floor playing with his kids when he suddenly collapsed. After a nurse explained about arrangements for her husband's body, I walked her outside to get her a cab. As we approached the curb, she turned and asked me, "How do I tell our two children that their Daddy isn't coming home?"

I've lived with that question every day since then. I talked with Roselle about it that evening when I got home, and in the years that followed came to understand that I would never have a good enough answer, for that patient's wife or for any of my other patients' loved ones. But if I became a cardiologist, I could work to reduce the number of times the question was asked.

Today I am the Director of the Urban Community Cardiology Program at the New York University School of Medicine in New York City and the Co-President of the Founders Affiliate of the American Heart Association (New York, New Jersey, Connecticut, Massachusetts, Maine, Vermont, Rhode Island, and New Hampshire). I spend a good deal of time developing programs, administering the department, and mentoring young physicians, but the most challenging and most rewarding part of my work is the time I devote each day to learning about my patients and from them, and using the experience and knowledge I have gained during my career to provide them with the

best possible medical care and the best possible strategies to outlive heart disease. What challenges me every day is crafting the
information from the new science and clinical studies that have
been published since my time as a resident into practical medical
strategies that keep heart disease a chronic condition rather than
a death sentence. These strategies include appropriate medications, diet, exercise, and "mind work" that I often prescribe for
my patients and which I describe in the pages of this book.

I've also learned from my own reactions to a disease to which
almost no one is immune, including cardiologists. During my
first year of training in my new specialty, I was assisting one of
the senior cardiologists in examining X-rays of the coronary
arteries of two young men whose only complaint had been chest
pain. In both cases we found extensive blockage, and both
patients were sent for immediate open-heart surgery. These two
men were hardly older than I was at the time. The next morning
I awoke with a racing heart that lasted almost 30 minutes, and
returned on and off throughout the day. It must be my nerves, I
thought, then wondered if that's what these two men had thought
as well. My racing, "jumping" heartbeat lasted for a whole week,
and ended only after I consulted a cardiologist, who assured me
that I was suffering from stress, not heart disease. But that day I
learned that heart disease is both a disease of the body *and* of
the mind, and that to prevent it, and even more crucially, to outlive it, we needed to address both aspects in our treatment.

Our knowledge today about what causes heart disease is light
years ahead of what we knew during my schooling (I graduated
medical school in 1967 and finished my cardiology training in
1974), and I devote the entire Introduction that follows to the
"New Science" involved in the way cardiology is practiced today.
Smoking was identified as a risk factor, clinically, only in the
mid-fifties, and wasn't recognized by the general public as such
until the late sixties. (The Surgeon General's famous warning

label on cigarette packages wasn't made mandatory until 1965, and television and radio cigarette advertising was banned in 1969. The package warning label did not mention heart disease risk until 1981.) In fact, many of the doctors with whom I worked, or by whom I was taught, were themselves heavy smokers and maintained that there was no connection between that nasty habit and heart disease. I remember spending many hours of my internship and residency at Downstate Medical School in Brooklyn poring over books in the Perrin-Long Library, named after one of the school's earliest chiefs of medicine, Dr. William Perrin-Long. Hanging over an ornate conference table in the main room of the library was an imposing portrait of the doctor, formally dressed in waistcoat and vest. It wasn't until after I'd chosen cardiology as my specialty that I finally noticed that in the good doctor's right hand, poised elegantly between two fingers, was a smoldering cigarette.

Our ignorance extended to other so-called lifestyle issues. The doctors who trained me were not convinced that fat and cholesterol had anything to do with atherosclerosis. Doing some sort of regular exercise was considered a good idea as a way to maintain overall health, but not because we knew of any direct connection between a sedentary lifestyle and the incidence of heart attack. Even after the famous Framingham study (see New Rule No. 2) began proving all these things to be determining risk factors of heart disease, doctors were reluctant to discuss behaviors such as smoking, diet, and exercise with their patients, or indeed to modify their own risky behaviors accordingly. Doctors, like everybody else, didn't want to give up their cigarettes and butter.

As dramatically as our understanding of heart disease has changed since the fifties, it pales in comparison to what we've learned just in the past five or ten years. I consider myself privileged to be a heart specialist during a time of such explosive growth and change in my field. We are making exciting break-throughs every month in the development of new and powerful drugs and interventions that have changed completely the way we prevent and treat America's greatest killer. At the same time, we've made important discoveries about the way we eat and play and work and the relationship to a healthy heart, and even the profound role that anger, stress, and social isolation play in how well we fare in attempting to beat this disease. What these discoveries have proved, in fact, is what we in the medical community had been suspecting for a long time and now have hard evidence to support: that *how* we live has a lot to do with *how long* we live. My original hope—to reduce the number of people who ask the question that the young widow asked me decades ago—is finally becoming a reality. Even if you already have heart disease, in many cases you can outlive it, but you need to change how you play the game.

A NEW SET OF RULES

How much has the playing field of heart disease prevention and treatment changed in the past decade or so? The best metaphor I can think of is a sports one. Imagine you are the manager of a major-league baseball team that's competing in the World Series. On the morning of the seventh and deciding game you receive a hand-delivered letter from the commissioner's office:

> *"Good Morning,"* it reads. *"Last night at a meeting of the commissioner and owners it was decided that the rules of baseball would be changed, EFFECTIVE IMMEDI-ATELY! The new rules are: 4 strikes to an out, 4 outs to an inning, and the center- and right-field walls will be moved in by 20 feet. Good luck in the game today."*

All of a sudden you have to rethink your entire strategy. Your previous star pitcher, who was good for five to seven innings, may now need to be replaced after three or four. And your average right-field hitter, whose long balls always fall just short of the wall, may suddenly be your new star home-run hitter. No time to argue about it—if you want to win, you need to adapt to the new rules!

In the last decade the rules for outliving heart disease—living well with your heart until you die of something else—have changed as dramatically for you and your doctors as they did for the baseball manager and his players. New scientific discoveries and a resulting new understanding of how heart disease develops have made this a time of incredible opportunity for those who suffer from cardiac illness and for those who are at risk in order to prevent it. And, unfortunately, that includes just about all of us.

Cardiovascular disease (heart disease and stroke) is still the number-one cause of death in the United States. More than half of us will actually die of heart disease or stroke, and many others will suffer its symptoms and disability. It becomes the chief cause of death in men starting at age 35 and of women at age 50. And more women between the ages of 40 and 50 will die of heart disease than breast cancer, despite a popular belief to the contrary. In fact, deaths from heart disease and stroke in the United States occur more frequently than deaths *from all forms of cancer combined!* In New York City alone, 28,000 people die each year of heart attacks and 22,000 suffer a stroke significant enough to require being hospitalized. And although those of us with inherited risk factors, such as diabetes or a family history of sudden heart attacks, are at greater risk from birth, the risk is there for all of us and increases as we age. In a sense, we are all "born to the game."

And that's where this book comes in. In it you'll find the very latest information available that's been proven to be meaningful and important on preventing and treating heart disease. That's not the same thing as seeing newspaper and magazine headlines day after day about "breakthroughs" that send us running to our doctors demanding the most recent techniques and treatment. Because it is a near universal health issue, the business of treating heart disease has grown into an enormous and lucrative industry. A great deal of new and confusing information about experimental findings is disseminated to the public every week, some of which is refuted within months when held up to closer scrutiny and properly controlled clinical testing. But when the chatter dies down, a very small percentage of that information *is* meaningful and crucial for you to have because it will affect not only how long you live, but how well you live each day. It is that information I want to share with you.

After a discussion of the New Science involved in preventing and treating heart disease, I lay out 10 chapters that each present a New Rule for beating heart disease that, in the last decade, has altered the way doctors treat patients. If you want to win, you need to take these new rules "to heart." They begin, simply enough, with ways of finding out whether or not you *have* heart disease and, if you do, how to get started on a program for managing your illness. We'll take a new look at risk factors and see what the current research shows about the impact that family history, high blood pressure, obesity, and smoking have on your heart health. We'll discuss the latest developments in statins and other heart drugs and talk about side effects and the importance of taking medicines as they are prescribed. Great strides have been made not only in surgical options, but in minor interventions that allow you to avoid major surgery. We'll take a fresh look at how diet and exercise affect heart health, and help you create a realistic plan you'll be able to stick with and see results from. We'll look at some of the truly exciting developments in the link between heart disease and our mental state, and sort out what helps and what doesn't in the complex world of alternative and complementary medicines. Finally, we'll discuss one of the most important issues in living well with heart disease: partnering with your doctors to ensure you're taking advantage of all that these new developments offer you, the patient.

For a number of years I've run a cardiac prevention program for people in the community through the 92nd Street Y, one of the largest cultural and educational institutions in New York. Several times a year I try to share with the hundreds of people present, in plain language, the latest developments that have been made in cardiology and how they can take advantage of this, starting *today*. They are terrific listeners and after my talk always have countless questions about this treatment or that drug. They are sometimes confused about something they read in the paper or something that did or did not work, for their uncle. While I can't answer even a fraction of their questions in the little time we have during these talks, I've done my best to share all that I know in this book. It is these people in my community, and the larger community of people I've treated over the last 28 years, who have taught me the most important lesson of all: that every day we outlive heart disease is a day worth living.

Introduction

THE NEW SCIENCE BEHIND THE NEW RULES
FOR OUTLIVING HEART DISEASE

The heart is a constantly working muscle that is fueled by the metabolism, or "burning," of fats and, in times of stress, sugars. These nutrients and the oxygen required to fuel the metabolism are supplied by the blood that courses though the heart's arteries—the coronary arteries. What is commonly referred to as "heart disease" is, in fact, a disease of these coronary arteries, hence the name coronary artery disease (also referred to as CAD).

Coronary artery disease will affect heart muscle when the arteries become blocked by accumulations of cholesterol and other material called plaque. Coronary artery disease is the reason for 98 percent of all heart attacks. Although it's our heart muscle that suffers when we develop this disease, the real focus of the "New Science" I describe is on the coronary arteries. This disease process that affects our arteries and ultimately our heart is called atherosclerosis and, in order to outlive heart disease, we need to dramatically change its pace and direction.

When I started my training as a cardiologist in the early

1970s, it would have been the height of folly to think that we would be able to do this. Researchers then were injecting a solution into the arteries that showed us, on an X-ray film, the inside of the blood vessels, called the lumen. When the lumen was narrowed, it was due to a plaque, and very narrowed areas meant very large plaques. We understood that the development of these plaques took place over a long time, and thought that they produced a heart attack by growing so large they almost entirely blocked the artery. At the time we thought that the final step in developing a heart attack was the formation of a blood clot in the small remaining open area of the artery. This clot shut off the blood supply to heart muscle. My professors taught us that plaque, which took years to develop, was probably irreversible, or at best would take years of medications, diet, and exercise to effect even slight improvement.

Then came studies, experiments, and discoveries that changed all of this thinking about heart disease. The "dream" of turning back heart disease became a goal, and is now a realistic goal. This New Science led to highly effective new lifestyle and treatment strategies that enable us today to prevent or outlive our heart disease. This New Science is the reason you and I can enter into this discussion about the "New Rules": if we observe them, we can, in many instances, indeed outlive our disease.

The changes in our knowledge and thinking about heart disease are very important to understand when working with the 10 New Rules that follow this chapter. For me, knowing *why* something must be done usually makes it more likely that it will be done. There is a veritable mountain of information, though, and so I am going to present the key facts in two parts. First, I will inform you of critical pieces of information that have changed our thinking about heart disease over the last couple of decades. I have found that looking at "what we thought *then*" and "what we know *now*" (or, more realistically, what we *think* we know now) is a good way to approach this important material. Then I will describe the workings of the disease—atherosclerosis—as we understand it today.

WHAT WE THOUGHT THEN AND WHAT WE KNOW (OR THINK WE KNOW) NOW

How does plaque form in our blood vessels?

Then: We thought that the cells that line the inside of the blood vessels, called endothelial cells, were a barrier to the movement of LDL ("bad") cholesterol into the wall of the artery. We assumed that the endothelial cell layer had to be injured—by toxins such as cigarette smoke, or by the force of blood that occurs with high blood pressure—for LDL to become lodged in the vessel wall and start a plaque.

Now: We know that LDL cholesterol, at sufficiently high levels in the blood, can move into the wall of the arteries without any previous injury. Studies at several medical centers in the 1980s showed that injecting one lab animal's LDL cholesterol into a healthy sibling would soon result in the second animal's uninjured blood vessels becoming saturated with the injected LDL. We also now know that when the LDL in our blood rises to a high enough level, the endothelial cells that line our blood vessels begin to function poorly—pushing the atherosclerotic disease further along.

The formation of plaque is key to our understanding of the development and treatment of heart disease. It is described in more detail later in this chapter.

What actually causes a heart attack?

Then: As I mentioned, we thought heart attacks were caused by a plaque that would grow so large that it would almost totally block the blood vessel; then a small clot would form to close the little space left between the top of the plaque and the opposite wall of the vessel. Blood flow down the coronary artery would be completely shut off and, as a result, the heart cells that were dependent on this blood would die. (The medical term for a heart attack is myocardial infarction, from the ancient Greek and Latin: *myo* and *cardia,* for "muscle" and "heart," and *infarct*, for "death.")

Now: We know that plaque size, in most cases, is not what determines whether or not we have a heart attack. In fact, more heart attacks occur at the site of small plaques, some too small to be seen when we take angiograms (X-rays of the coronary arteries). What causes a heart attack is a clot, called a thrombus, that forms at a place where the surface of a plaque has broken open, or fractured. We've learned from patients who had angiograms some time prior to their heart attacks that heart attacks are frequently caused by fracture of a small plaque. From these angiograms, we learned that heart attack risk depends not on how big the plaque is but on how likely—or vulnerable—the plaque is to fracture.

Does bypass surgery (often called "CABG," for coronary artery bypass graft) prevent or reduce the chances of having a heart attack?

Then: CABG surgery was performed to create a bypass for blood to get around the blockage caused by a large plaque in one or more of the heart's coronary arteries. It was initially assumed that this procedure would prevent a heart attack if and when that large plaque grew to totally occlude the coronary artery.

Now: We found that patients who underwent bypass surgery for severe blockages in most or all of the coronary arteries lived longer than patients who were treated medically, that is, with drugs (such as statins) but no surgery. Interestingly, though, the surgical patients had the *same number* of heart attacks but successful surgery allowed them to survive more of their heart attacks than the group treated medically. In most circumstances, surgery was the right choice, since the patient lived longer; however, the disease that forms the plaque—atherosclerosis—continued to progress.

Could we "regress" coronary artery disease by lowering cholesterol levels and essentially turn back the clock on the amount of atherosclerosis in our vessels?

Then: Physicians knew that LDL cholesterol was produced in the liver and that patients with high LDL were more likely to have advanced atherosclerosis. They theorized that if LDL in the bloodstream could be lowered, patients would not form as many plaques and could shrink, or "regress," the plaques that they already had.

A major breakthrough in the lowering of the LDL level came with the introduction of lovastatin (Mevacor), the first of a class

---

Drugs are commonly referred to by their generic name first, followed by their well-known branded or patented name in parentheses, for example, lovastatin (Mevacor); atorvastatin (Lipitor). That form is followed in this book.

---

of drugs called statins, which inhibit a critical step in the liver for the body's production of LDL cholesterol. Statins allowed physicians, for the first time, to safely reduce LDL cholesterol by almost one-half in the overwhelming majority of patients. The pharmaceutical and medical communities saw this as a potential opportunity to restore a patient's arteries to a much lower level of disease, with fewer and smaller obstructing plaques. A series of studies, including the Familial Atherosclerosis Treatment Study (FATS) in the United States, was performed in the 1980s, and the results were published in 1990. Patients with coronary heart disease were enrolled in the study after plaques were seen on their angiograms. They were then randomly assigned to take a statin or a placebo. Cholesterol levels were monitored and angiograms were repeated at the end of a year and compared with the first ones to see if the plaques had progressed (that is, enlarged), stayed the same, or regressed. (At that time, there was no convincing clinical evidence that lowering cholesterol with statins would change clinical outcome and so it was still considered ethical to treat a group of patients with placebo.)

Now: The before-and-after angiograms were disappointing to the researchers. There was some evidence that more plaques regressed and fewer progressed in the statin patients than in the placebo patients. However, the amount of regression was very small, in the 2 to 4 percent range, hardly statistically significant, especially when computer-assisted techniques for measuring them could differ among skilled observers by as much as 5 percent!

But far more impressive was the *clinical outcome* of the patients in the statin and placebo groups. Over the one year that angiograms did not dramatically change, heart attacks, sudden cardiac death, and hospital admissions for bypass surgery dropped in the statin patients by a full one-third or more! In the

FATS trial, the group of patients who received lovastatin (Meva-cor) (to lower LDL) and the vitamin niacin (known to raise HDL) had more than a 75 percent reduction in clinical events over the untreated group.

These results "changed the rules" for winning the battle against heart disease, and the term "clinical regression" was coined for this effect, since "angiographic regression" was not seen in these studies.

What's the function of the endothelial cells that line the inside of our arteries?

Then: This layer of cells was thought of as a simple barrier that separated the factors in our blood that form a clot from a sub-stance in the wall of the artery called tissue factor, which would start the clotting process. This separation formed by the endothelial cell layer is important. We want a clot to form to help stop the bleeding if an artery is cut or torn, but we don't want a clot that will block the flow of blood to form inside an intact artery.

Now: The real importance of the endothelial cells that line the inside surface of our arteries was first brought to light by an experiment that won its creator a well-deserved Nobel Prize. In 1980 Dr. Robert Furshgott made a "rule-changing" discovery while working in a laboratory at the State University of New York Downstate Medical Center in Brooklyn, just down the hall from what was my office where I served as Chief of Cardi-ology. He prepared a strip of the wall of the major artery, the aorta, from a laboratory rabbit and suspended it in a saltwater bath to sustain it and keep it alive. To this strip he attached a gauge to measure its tension. When he added adrenalin to the bath, the tension would increase just as it would in the body:

the adrenalin caused the muscle cells in the aorta's wall to contract. When he added a chemical called acetylcholine, used by the nerves and other cells, the strip would relax almost back to the pre-adrenalin level, just as it would in our bodies.

In one instance, however, adding the acetylcholine didn't work and the strip remained contracted and its tension remained high. The reason that the acetylcholine didn't work as it had in all his prior experiments intrigued Dr. Furshgott and he carefully investigated how the aorta strips had been prepared for this experiment. He identified the difference. In this one experiment his laboratory technician, in preparing the strips, had worn a pair of gloves that were abrasive and had actually stripped off most of the endothelial cell layer from the aortic strip.

Dr. Furshgott then did a series of experiments with and without the endothelial cell layer on the aorta strip and he found that *only* when the endothelial cell layer was intact did he get the aorta to relax when acetylcholine was added. The reason was that a chemical substance in the endothelial cell layer that is released caused the blood vessel to relax. He first called this chemical EDRF—endothelium derived relaxation factor—and then, with other researchers, found that it is a molecule (one nitrogen, one oxygen) called nitric oxide (NO).

Suddenly, with one experiment, the endothelial cells were recognized, not as a passive barrier, but as a unique organ. When appropriately stimulated, these cells would produce substances with far-reaching effects on the body. We now know that these cells are the "control room" for coronary artery health and disease. They produce or are acted upon by over 60 chemicals and that they control, to a large extent, the development of atherosclerotic disease in the wall of the blood vessel and, in the case of a plaque, how vulnerable it is to fracture and cause a heart attack. The endothelial cell is a target of important new strategies in our battle to outlive heart disease.

What is the relationship between depression and heart disease?

Then: There was no reason to think that there was any connection between our mind or our feelings and the development of unstable plaques that led to atherosclerosis and heart attacks.

Now: There is now good evidence that tells us how the mind and emotions are linked to the health of our heart vessels! Negative emotional states, such as depression, anger, and social isolation, are important factors in the first and second heart attacks of many people! Large prospective studies have confirmed that depression is a powerful *predictor* of the development of coronary heart disease and cardiac events.

Today we know that heart patients who become depressed after developing the disease are significantly more likely to die from their heart disease than patients who are not depressed. A study of men with heart disease in Finland that was completed in the 1990s measured a combination of negative emotional factors that included anger, depression, and anxiety (sometimes referred to as the "distress emotions") and, together with an assessment of the presence or absence of social coping skills, arrived at what investigators termed a measurement of "type D personality." The investigators found a 4.7-fold increase in cardiac events in men with an elevated type D score.

HOW PLAQUE DEVELOPS IN OUR BLOOD VESSELS

The next change in our scientific knowledge that is the basis for new strategies to prevent and treat coronary artery disease is our understanding of the disease process, atherosclerosis, that results in plaque development. Plaques are collections of cholesterol, cells, and other substances that grow as bumps on the inside of our blood vessel walls. Our understanding of this process is not yet complete, but the current information allows me to explain it as five steps:

Step 1: Accumulation of LDL
Step 2: Oxidation of LDL
Step 3: Formation of Macrophage "Foam Cells"
Step 4: Inflammation of the Plaque
Step 5: Rupture of the Plaque

Step 1: Formation of LDL

We need some cholesterol to coat the connecting parts of our nerve cells and to make the hormones that regulate our growth and almost all of our important body functions. The cholesterol, the majority of it in the form of LDL, is mostly made in our liver (only about 20 percent is from the food we eat) and transported in our blood from there to the cells that need it. Too much LDL cholesterol in our blood, however, is a starting point for atherosclerosis, as the excess crosses over the layer of endothelial cells

Structure of Normal Coronary Artery

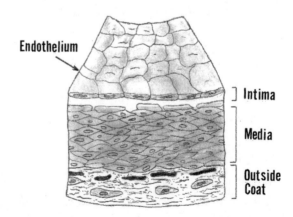

Endothelium

] Intima

] Media

] Outside Coat

that line the inside of our blood vessels to the "intimal" layer of our arteries and there begins the process that results in the development and growth of plaques.

Step 2: Oxidation of LDL

The next step in the process is the pivotal one leading to heart disease. The LDL that has moved inside that wall of the artery is mostly inactive and won't start atherosclerosis unless it is oxidized by "free radicals" that live in all of our tissues. Although this process sounds as if oxygen is involved, this oxidation is actually the transfer of very small electrically charged particles from atom to atom.

A word about free radicals: they are produced when our muscle cells metabolize sugars and fats to produce the high-energy adenosine triphosphate (also known as ATP), which fuels all of our physical work and bodily functions. So we can't stop this process. But while we constantly produce free radicals, our bodies are diligently rounding them up and neutralizing them with our bodies' chemicals (one of which is called superoxide desmutase, or SOD). When we produce more free radicals than we can neutralize, the process of oxidation in our bodies increases. In

Early Atherosclerotic Plaque Development

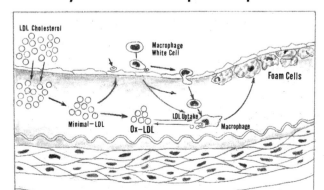

the case of the LDL cholesterol in the walls of our arteries, more of it is oxidized, jump-starting the atherosclerotic disease.

The oxidized LDL does this by initiating a series of events that results in the release of small chemicals, called cytokines, that bring even more LDL cholesterol and, of great importance, more white blood cells into the arterial wall.

Step 3: Formation of Macrophage "Foam Cells"

The white blood cells attracted into the wall of the artery are called macrophages, and they now proceed to ingest as much of the oxidized LDL cholesterol as they can. These macrophages that are full of oxidized LDL particles look a little like the foamy head on a glass of beer and are thus called foam cells. Foam cells are essential to atherosclerosis and can only be made from oxidized LDL cholesterol particles, because the macrophage won't ingest "normal" LDL cholesterol. The foam cells produce the cytokines and other chemicals that create the next stage of atherosclerosis—inflammation. They also explain why a plaque has

Advanced Atherosclerotic Plaque with Rupture

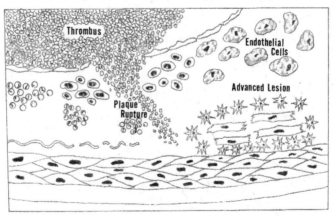

a soft center of cholesterol: the foam cells gradually move to the center of the plaque, where they break apart and release their cholesterol particles.

Step 4: Inflammation of the Plaque

Foam cells and endothelial cells release more cytokines to keep the growth process going and the plaque now looks very similar to, and shares important characteristics with, any area of infection or reaction to a foreign agent—for instance, the red and painful area in your skin that forms around a splinter embedded in your finger. This process is called inflammation and at this stage the atherosclerotic plaque is described as inflammatory. The foam cells gather at the edge, or shoulder, of the plaque (where it joins the more normal arterial wall), and begin to secrete an enzyme that can dissolve the collagen in the cap of the arterial plaque.

Coronary Artery Atherosclerotic Plaque in Acute Myocardial Infarction

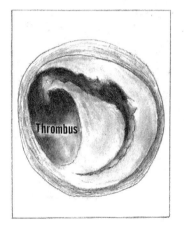

Step 5: Rupture of the Plaque

The cap is critical to the containment of a plaque. When it starts to weaken, the plaque can rupture, leading to a life-threatening blood clot. The final step consists of the changes in the plaque that lead to its fracture. Plaques that are susceptible to fracture are called vulnerable plaques and can become the site of heart attack-causing thrombi.

When we look at them under a microscope, vulnerable plaques have four characteristics that differentiate them from other plaques: (1) a larger amount of cholesterol at the center of the plaque, (2) more "foam cells" in the plaque and especially around the edges of the plaque, (3) a thinner tissue cap over the inner surface of the plaque, and (4) fewer smooth muscle cells throughout the plaque. The latter three differences are connected, because it's the smooth muscle cells in a plaque that produce collagen fibers. These fibers give the cap strength and substance. This strength is attacked by the foam cells, which produce special enzymes (named metaloproteinases) that dissolve collagen and can weaken the cap.

The importance of plaque vulnerability can be appreciated when we note that plaques that rupture in blood vessels to the heart cause heart attacks.

NEW SCIENCE AND THE NEW RULES

This new scientific knowledge that has enabled us to more fully understand heart disease and the process of atherosclerosis is the basis for the new strategies that I think of as the New Rules for outliving heart disease. These rules, outlined in the following chapters, have made possible my dream of helping my patients, my family, and myself to outlive heart disease—and I now share them with you:

My 10 New Rules for outliving heart disease are:

1. **Know** if you have heart disease, or, more critically, whether you are having a heart attack.

2. **Identify** your risk factors—old and new—for developing heart disease.
3. **Include** statins: learn about these and similar wonder drugs and why they prevent coronary events.
4. **Establish** and maintain an exercise program: know why exercise is so important.
5. **Select and stick to** the best diet for your heart.
6. **Reduce** stress, anxiety, anger, and depression.
7. **Explore** alternative and complementary medical treatment.
8. **Keep up** with the latest diagnostic, medical, pharmaceutical, and surgical therapies in treating heart disease.
9. **Understand** how your heritage may alter your heart disease risk: a special word for African Americans, Hispanics, and others.
10. **Partner** with your doctor to establish and reach your health goals by working together for a winning program: determine together strategies for risk reduction and outliving heart disease.

I have chosen to present in these pages the new knowledge and the resulting new strategies as the 10 New Rules you need to know to outlive heart disease. The following chapters explain how to determine and understand your risk of developing heart disease and how to apply all the new knowledge, medications, and lifestyle choices in order to outlive it.

BE ALERT TO SYMPTOMS THAT SIGNAL IMMINENT HEART ATTACK

One of my most valued colleagues early in my career was a brilliant MD and PhD nuclear medicine specialist. At the time he and I were working to develop a program of nuclear isotope cardiac stress testing at the medical school. Nat demonstrated on a daily basis the value of thinking critically and carefully about the images we were producing in our patients. The last real conversation I had with him was at 5:30 in the afternoon when he sat in my office and asked me to look at an electrocardiogram he had carried with him all day. He had done it on himself after awakening with chest pain, for the first time, that morning. It showed a large area of damaged heart muscle and he was immediately admitted to our coronary care unit—14 hours after his chest pain began. He died there that evening. With today's new science and new techniques, prompt medical care would have greatly increased his chance of outliving his heart disease.

• • •

The greatest risk of dying of heart disease is not realizing you have it, so the first New Rule for outliving it is to be aware of symptoms, conditions, and aspects of your family health history that indicate you may need immediate treatment or evaluation. This chapter offers the information you need to make the decisions that could save your life.

Many of us have heart disease, but don't know it until we first begin to experience life-threatening symptoms, symptoms which are, at first, often ignored. Fully half of heart attacks or sudden cardiac deaths occur in men and women who did not even know they had heart disease. One-quarter of these victims die—most before they reach the hospital emergency room. All of the technological and scientific advances in treating heart disease that we've made in recent years, which are discussed in succeeding chapters, mean nothing if a person doesn't know he or she is at high risk and needs to get—quickly!—the best care available. A sad but telling statistic is that the incidence of sudden cardiac death (usually defined as death within one hour of the first symptom) has stayed the same over the past 10 years, despite an impressive reduction in the overall death rate from heart disease.

To complicate this situation further, symptoms of the onset of a heart attack may differ between men and women (see pages 49–52). Family history of heart disease may affect men and women at different ages. Your racial and cultural profile may affect the likelihood of a sudden cardiac event at an earlier age than what you may think of as the "norm." What's the "norm"? Before the mid-1990s, virtually all studies of heart disease were done on white *men*. So the data and information arising from those studies are what your doctor and his medical team were taught in medical school. Since the mid-90s, when the National Institutes of Health mandated it, women have been included in all clinical heart studies, but in some cases the data are still too new to be commonly known by health care professionals or are inconclusive and need further study. (For instance, a baby aspirin taken daily appears to have different effects in men and women regarding heart attack and stroke prevention. The most recent studies indicate that aspirin prevents heart attacks only in women who already have heart disease.)

Therefore, if you are a woman, you need to be particularly aware that you might experience symptoms other than the ones generally recognized in men as those that indicate a sudden heart attack or a need for immediate evaluation to prevent an attack. The information you need is given in more detail in New Rule No. 9 (beginning on page 203).

To determine if you have heart disease and need immediate evaluation, take the following steps:

LISTEN TO YOUR BODY

It may be hard to accept but, if you are like most people, your first impulse when you feel something different and concerning in your body is to deny that anything is wrong. Even if we experience symptoms that many of us recognize as dangerous, such as pressing chest pain going to the jaw or left arm that occurs during stress or activity, we may try to ignore how we're feeling or assign the symptoms to other causes ("I moved some boxes yesterday so my chest is sore" or "Must be that spicy food I had for dinner!").

If this behavior "rings true," you are not alone. In my experience, some of the worst offenders, and thus the victims in this regard, are doctors and nurses. My colleague, Nat, is an example.

When you combine our ingrained sense of denial with the fact that first symptoms, especially in women, patients with diabetes, or those of us over 65 years of age, are often similar to those of temporary gastrointestinal problems (note the name—

heartburn), fatigue, anxiety, or a viral "flu," it is easy to understand how so many of us ignore the signals. Listening to your body is the first step in learning if you have heart disease, and thus the first step in your strategy to outlive it.

KNOW THE SYMPTOMS THAT INDICATE A HEART ATTACK MAY BE IMMINENT

Here is my list of symptoms and feelings that indicate you have to be evaluated and tested. Most of us will have some of these symptoms. The more you have, the more recently they have occurred, and the more related they are to exercise or emotional stress, the more important they are. Although in many instances the cause of these symptoms will not be heart disease, the risk that they are is too great to ignore!

- Chest sensations that include dull, pressing feelings or pain that are initiated with emotional stress or physical activity. When these are relieved by rest, or with a nitroglycerin tablet under the tongue (whether prescribed or provided by a first responder/emergency medical technician), they frequently indicate a diagnosis of angina pectoris (chest pain caused by disease in the arteries that supply the heart with blood). This indicates that you have coronary artery atherosclerosis with a plaque in your coronary artery that narrows the inside space and restricts the flow of blood to the heart muscle.
- Similar sensations that you feel in your shoulder or arm (usually the left one, but not always) or jaw.
- Abdominal pain, pressure, or burning with exercise or stress.
- Repeatedly feeling weak, profoundly fatigued, nause-

ated, dizzy, near faint or fainting with exercise or stress or at rest.

- Shortness of breath during exercise that is greater than the given amount of exercise usually evokes.

A Note to Women about Symptoms of Heart Disease

Over the last 5 to 10 years, we have learned that women are more likely than men to have "atypical" symptoms of heart disease or imminent heart attack. Therefore, if you are a woman, you may experience any of these "typical" symptoms, but you may also experience other symptoms that indicate you need immediate evaluation by a health care professional, preferably in an emergency room setting. Heart disease or heart attack symptoms in women may include:

- Persistent burning or sharp pains in the chest or abdomen
- Indigestion that is not relieved by antacids
- Strong feelings of fatigue, shortness of breath, nausea
- Unexplained perspiration
- Periods of fast heartbeat

Unless these symptoms can be explained by another reason known to you (for instance, menopausal flushes, an infection, or a drug side effect), they should alert you to the fact that you need to seek medical attention for possible heart disease. See New Rule No. 9 (beginning on page 203) for more information about women and heart disease.

Important: If these symptoms occur at rest or with exercise and remain more than a few minutes after exercise or stress, or if they are new, and especially if they make you anxious or fearful, then you should go to the closest hospital emergency room. These symptoms could be of no real consequence or they could be the beginning of a heart attack or an intermediate condition called unstable coronary syndrome, which has a real chance of progressing to a heart attack. With immediate and excellent care in a hospital setting, the heart attack can often be prevented. If it is already under way, good immediate care can limit the amount of damage to your heart muscle. If you stay at home or at work waiting and worrying about these symptoms, they can develop into a full-fledged heart attack and increase your risk of dying!

SYMPTOMS OF IMMINENT HEART ATTACK IN MEN

- Crushing chest pain
- Pain in other areas of upper body (arms, back, neck, jaw, stomach)
- Shortness of breath, cold sweat, nausea, light-headedness
- Fatigue
- Less commonly, the symptoms noted below

SYMPTOMS OF IMMINENT HEART ATTACK IN WOMEN

- **One or all** of the above symptoms, **or**
- Pain or discomfort in the center of the chest or abdomen
- Pain or discomfort in other areas of upper back (arms, back, neck, jaw, stomach)
- Indigestion unrelieved by antacids
- Diffuse or transient feelings of nausea, vomiting, shortness of breath, light-headedness, sleeplessness, racing heartbeat
- Unusual or unexplained perspiration
- Back and/or jaw pain

Most of the information we have about heart disease comes from observation and studies of Caucasian men that began after World War II, when the incidence of heart disease in women was thought to be very low. What scientists have discovered in the last decade is that most women who develop heart disease do so after menopause, about 10 years later than men do, and their symptoms can be quite different from men's and therefore overlooked. For these reasons, most women are not tested or screened for heart disease as rigorously as men are. It is important for postmenopausal women to demand cardiac screening, especially if they are having symptoms that could point the way to heart disease.

Heart disease is the leading cause of death in American women; it is *six times* more deadly than breast cancer. Why? In part because symptoms differ from men's, women are not screened as rigorously, and their disease is caught at a much later stage, when treatment options may be limited.

KNOW YOUR GENERAL MEDICAL CONDITION AND NOTE FAMILY HISTORY

The next question to ask yourself is whether you have a medical condition or a disease that makes it very likely that you also have heart disease. (Refer to New Rule No. 9, beginning on page 203, for more information.) In some instances the medical condition or disease will reflect advanced atherosclerosis, the basis of most heart disease. In other instances, the condition will be tied directly to factors (such as high blood pressure) that promote atherosclerosis. In many families with early heart disease in the parents, the cause is not known but the risk to the children is apparent.

The following is the **list of medical conditions** that make it likely that coronary artery disease is present; if you display these conditions, testing for heart disease is advisable, even if you are not experiencing acute symptoms of imminent heart attack.

- *Adult-onset diabetes (also known as diabetes mellitus or type II diabetes).* In those who develop diabetes in adulthood and require treatment either with pills or insulin, coronary artery disease occurs more than twice as often as in the general population. This risk is further increased if diabetes is associated with other risk factors such as high cholesterol, high blood pressure, and obesity. By an overwhelming margin, the number-one cause of death in most adults with diabetes is heart disease or stroke.

- *Clinical conditions due to atherosclerosis in other arteries,* such as stroke or peripheral vascular disease (atherosclerosis in the arteries that carry the blood to the legs), greatly increase your chance of having coronary artery atherosclerosis as well and therefore the risk of a heart attack.

- *Strong family history in a person at the appropriate age.* If you have one or more primary relatives, that is, a parent, brother, or sister who developed coronary disease at a young age (before 55 in male relatives and 65 in female relatives), you must pay attention to your own risk of developing heart disease. In some instances, the absence of an additional major risk factor (for example, your parent smoked and you have not, or your parent or sibling had a very high LDL cholesterol and you do not) will clearly lower your risk, compared to your parent or sibling with coronary heart disease. Testing still may be a reasonable approach for you. In my patients this testing usually occurs when they get anxious as they approach the date of a parent's heart attack or death—this is often referred to as an "anniversary reaction"—but testing optimally should be done well before this age if you are to optimize your chances to outlive heart disease!

If you are experiencing symptoms of acute heart disease, do not succumb to denial. Go directly to the nearest hospital emergency room for immediate evaluation and possible treatment. If you are a woman, you may have to be assertive about having a cardiac evaluation, since your symptoms may differ from those that are well known to the emergency room staff to be heart disease. If you are diabetic or have a primary relative who developed heart disease or died from it at a young age, you need to do two things: (1) make an appointment with your doctor for further evaluation (see New Rule No. 10: Partner with Your Doctor to Reach Your Heart-Health Goals, beginning on page 230), and (2) read the next chapter, which goes into detail about assessing your risk factors for developing heart disease in the next 10 years.

Let me reinforce the goal of this book, which is to *prevent* heart disease, or if you already have it, to *manage* your heart disease so it becomes a chronic condition, not a terminal event. In order for you to be successful in this goal, you need to arm yourself with as much information as possible about the disease itself and the likelihood you'll develop it. The next New Rule for outliving heart disease invites you to assess your risk factors for having a heart attack.

KNOW YOUR RISK FOR HAVING A HEART ATTACK IN THE NEXT 10 YEARS

If you are not diabetic, have no first-order relatives (that is, mom, dad, brother, sister) who developed or died from heart disease in the prime of life, and are experiencing no symptoms, can you assume you are free of coronary disease? Unfortunately, the answer is NO! New Rule No. 2 for outliving heart disease outlines the risk factors doctors use for determining if a patient is likely to develop heart disease within the next 10 years. The information in this chapter will lead you through the doctor's evaluation process so that you can discuss with your own physician your risk of coronary disease. This self-evaluation process takes into account the most important heart disease risk factors and is a tool to address the question of what your actual risk is.

BACKGROUND: THE SEVEN COUNTRIES STUDY AND THE FRAMINGHAM STUDY

Much of the valuable information about heart disease risk factors was gathered from 1958 to 1970, when an international inquiry, known as the Seven Countries Study, was conducted in populations of men ages 40 to 59. The inquiry studied the death rates from heart disease in seven countries (Yugoslavia, Italy, Greece, Finland, the Netherlands, the United States, and Japan) that were selected because of the availability of valid death certificates and because they represented differences in racial and ethnic populations, the structure of society and economy (industrial versus farming), and diets. (For a more detailed discussion of the diets that prevail in each country and their effects on each country's rate of heart disease, see New Rule No. 5, beginning on page 96.) Comparison of cardiac death rates within each society and between societies noted a correlation between heart disease and smoking, hypertension, and blood cholesterol levels, and suggested the importance of daily physical work and diet. The profound increase in heart death rates in northern European countries (Finland, the Netherlands) when compared to Mediterranean (Italy, Greece) and Pacific Rim (Japan) countries laid the groundwork for what is considered the single most important study in heart attack prevention—the Framingham Heart Study.

In 1949 scientists from the Boston medical schools selected Framingham, Massachusetts, for a long-range study that would address the influence of known and unknown factors associated with heart disease. A stable community, where the population and the health care systems were willing to participate, was critical to this choice. The initial group of more than 5,200 adults (2,336 men and 2,873 women) underwent a comprehensive series of exams, interviews, and blood tests (including blood serum samples that were frozen for testing at a later date, as additional tests became relevant and available). These subjects were then re-evaluated every second year, and events such as the onset of angina pectoris, heart attacks, sudden death, and, more recently, bypass surgery, angioplasty, and stenting were noted. Since 1972, in order to more fully determine the role of familial and genetic factors in the onset of heart disease, many of the children of the original group underwent full medical evaluations and are now re-examined every four years.

The first "look-back" analysis took place seven years after the original study began, when patients who had heart-related events described above were analyzed to find out what they had in common in their initial evaluation that was different when compared with others in this population who did not have such events. The group that had experienced some sort of heart event during the follow-up period was statistically more likely to have initially had the following findings in their charts:

- Elevated blood cholesterol levels
- Elevated blood pressure
- Cigarette smoking

The Framingham study termed these items "major risk factors" for developing heart disease. To be considered a major risk factor, an item had to meet the following criteria:

- It was *uniquely important* in determining heart attack risk (as is the case with blood pressure).
- It *increased the risk as it increased in level;* that is, risk was greater if the person's cholesterol was 350 as compared to 250, or if the person smoked two packs of cigarettes a day rather than one pack a day.
- Each was *additive,* meaning that if the person smoked two packs of cigarettes a day, his or her heart attack risk was higher if blood pressure was 180/90 than it was if it was the normal value of 120/80. The blood pressure risk is *added to* the cigarette risk!

As the study progressed, other risk factors were added to the "major" list:

- Adult-onset diabetes, also known as type II or diabetes mellitus, which usually starts in adulthood and can be controlled, initially at least, by pills instead of insulin injections
- Obesity
- Sedentary lifestyle; that is, not being at least moderately active for a minimum of 30 minutes per day
- Metabolic syndrome—a particularly high-risk combination of obesity, high blood pressure, low HDL ("good" cholesterol), high triglycerides, and early signs of diabetes

The Framingham study has now exceeded its fifty-fifth year and has been continually funded by the National Institutes of Health. It has more than paid for itself by virtue of a continued output of new information regarding the prevention of heart disease. Repeated examinations of the children of the original Framingham group, the addition to the study group of a neighboring population to address risk factors in African Americans, and the remarkable ability to do new blood assays on serum frozen up to 40 years ago have essentially "written the book" on heart disease risk factors.

Other important risk factors have emerged from the Framingham study and from other studies. These include:

- Depression
- Elevated levels of certain blood chemicals, including homocysteine (an amino acid that promotes plaque in the arteries); C-reactive protein (CRP) (a protein that

indicates inflammation in the body), and lipoprotein, or Lp(a) (a blood particle that may promote plaque growth and clotting)

These risk factors not only allow doctors to estimate a person's risk of dying of heart disease over a 10-year period, but also prompt them to look for atherosclerosis (the buildup of plaque in the blood vessels described in the Introduction). These risk factors are the target of medications and interventions aimed at preventing and decreasing the progression of the disease. A critical part of the New Rules for outliving heart disease program, they are described below and more fully addressed in later chapters where specific strategies to outlive heart disease are discussed in detail.

THE CHOLESTEROL-RELATED FACTORS THAT PREDICT YOUR HEART ATTACK RISK

Cholesterol is a molecule that the body uses for multiple purposes, two of which are lining the membranes around cells and serving as a building block for hormones and other substances essential to life. "Cholesterol," when used as a generic term, refers to the group of particles of cholesterol and fats that travel in the bloodstream. These particles are both absorbed in the bloodstream as we digest our food and manufactured by the liver and circulated by our bloodstream. They are packaged in a coating of protein so that they dissolve in our blood plasma and do not form the droplets we would see if we dripped oil into a jar of water. Hence the name "lipoprotein" is used to refer to the different cholesterol and fat-containing particles.

There are three separate groups of particles that, along with total cholesterol (the sum of cholesterol in all the lipoprotein particles), are reported in a "lipid profile" that we get as part of a blood test and that indicates our risk of developing atherosclerosis. These are:

- Low-density lipoprotein cholesterol particles (LDL cholesterol)
- High-density lipoprotein cholesterol particles (HDL cholesterol)
- Triglycerides (particles made up of a small sugarlike molecule and three attached fatty acid molecules)

All three of these particles, if they are present in abnormal levels (elevated in the case of LDL and triglycerides, and reduced in the case of HDL cholesterol), are understood to increase the risk of atherosclerosis and consequent heart attacks and strokes. The numbers for lipoproteins are given as mg/dl, that is, weight in milligrams of the particles per one-tenth of a liter (abbreviated "dl") of blood serum. As a reference range (I will discuss specific goals for lipoprotein levels later in this chapter), "good" levels of the lipoproteins for patients with heart disease or significant increased risk (as in patients with diabetes) are less than

The reason for the two values for LDL cholesterol (70mg/dl and 100mg/dl) as being "good" for people with heart disease or with increased risk factors is that the guidelines are in transition. A number of studies show that lowering LDL to 70 instead of 100 will further reduce heart disease progression and heart attacks, but the number of people studied is still relatively small, compared with the studies that show the benefit of getting to below 100mg/dl. At present, the guidelines for doctors read that the physician can, "as an option," reduce LDL cholesterol in this group of patients below 70mg/dl. This is an option I almost always take!

200mg/dl for total cholesterol and less than 100mg/dl or 70mg/dl for LDL cholesterol, less than 150mg/dl for triglycerides, and greater than 45mg/dl in men and greater than 55mg/dl in women for HDL cholesterol.

Elevated total cholesterol in the blood is a marker of increased risk and was the lipoprotein measured in the first Framingham analysis. Recent studies have indicated that the LDL cholesterol, the major contributor to the total cholesterol measurement, is the most predictive of risk. The Multiple Risk Factor Intervention Trial, known as MRFIT, is another large study with multiyear data collection. This study, which began in 1971, showed that a total cholesterol of 250mg/dl was associated with nearly four times the risk of a heart attack over the six-year study period, as was a total cholesterol level of 180mg/dl, and made lipid reduction the cornerstone therapy for preventing and treating heart disease. New knowledge of the specifics of this relationship and new drugs and strategies to modify these lipid levels are the basis of an important New Rule for outliving heart disease.

Although total and LDL cholesterol are major predictors of risk, it is important to remember that 20 percent of heart attacks in the Framingham study have been in men in whom total and LDL cholesterol were in the normal or near-normal range. Studies have further divided these LDL cholesterol particles on the basis of size and density into four subtypes, and the evidence indicates that the smaller and denser the LDL particles are, the more atherogenic (that is, most able to promote plaque development in blood vessels), and thus represent the greatest risk to the patient.

HDL cholesterol is, in contrast to LDL cholesterol, "cardio-protective" and inversely related to the risk of suffering a heart attack. The higher a person's blood level of HDL cholesterol, the lower is his or her risk, while a low HDL level represents a major risk factor for coronary heart disease. Framingham data show that for a person with moderately elevated LDL cholesterol, an HDL level in the high range results in one-quarter the risk of heart attack when compared with a person with the same LDL reading and an HDL level in the lowest range. When HDL levels were related to heart attack in the Framingham population, a 1mg/dl increase in HDL was associated with a 2 percent reduction in heart attack risk in men and a 3 percent reduction in women.

Triglycerides, the lipoproteins made up of the sugar molecule glycerol and three fatty acid molecules, were initially thought not to be a risk factor for heart attacks, but recent analysis of clinical data from the Framingham population and elsewhere indicates that it does predict heart attack risk. This is especially so when high triglycerides are present in patients who have central obesity (defined as a waist measurement greater than 40 inches in men or 35 inches in women), and other symptoms of metabolic syndrome (being overweight; having low HDL lipoproteins, high triglycerides, and high blood pressure; and having elevated fasting blood sugar). Patients with this syndrome are resistant to the effect of their own insulin, which, in turn, forces the body to produce greater amounts of it. At high levels, insulin promotes atherosclerosis. The syndrome, often an early sign of diabetes, is associated with a very significant increase in coronary heart disease risk. The dramatic increase in obesity in the United States and the associated rise in diabetes reflect this relationship. Without a national program to reduce obesity by dietary changes and increased physical activity, metabolic syndrome will cause a dramatic increase in heart disease in the next generation—our children.

BEYOND FRAMINGHAM

Every three to seven years a committee of scientists, health care providers, and epidemiologists from a variety of disciplines and representing major government agencies and professional organizations reviews the recent data from clinical studies and publishes the range of each of the lipoproteins that are considered best for people at the low-, intermediate-, and high-risk levels of developing heart disease, as well as the treatment goal levels for different groups of patients. This committee, the Adult Treatment Panel of the National Cholesterol Education Program (NCEP ATP), also recommends specific treatments. The past several guidelines issued by the panel have decreased the level of "normal," or low-risk cholesterol and LDL cholesterol, as data was accumulated that show improvement in patient outcomes with treatment to lower lipoproteins levels. Thus, a person with an LDL cholesterol level who was told 10 years ago that it was fine may be told today that his or her level is too high and requires treatment to lower it.

The following are the current (revised in 2004) NCEP ATP guidelines for physicians regarding lipoproteins (mg/dl):

LDL Cholesterol

<70	An "optional level" of choice for patients with heart disease who are at high risk
<100	Optimal
100–129	Near Optimal/Above Optimal
130–159	Borderline High
160–189	High
>190	Very High

Total Cholesterol

<200	Desirable
200–239	Borderline High
>240	High

HDL Cholesterol

<40	Low
>60	High

Triglycerides

<150	Normal
150–199	Borderline High
200–499	High
>500	Very High

The LDL "goal levels" are set according to the number of other risk factors a person has, such as cigarette smoking, high blood pressure, a low HDL (<40), a family history of coronary heart disease in a first-order relative under the age 55 for a male relative and 65 for a female relative, and the age of the patient (over 45 years for men and over 55 years for women). The guidelines are as follows:

Risk Category	LDL Goal (mg/dl)
Coronary heart disease (already) or "risk equivalent" such as diabetes	<70 or <100
Two or more risk factors (or one if over age 45 in men and 55 in women)	<130
Zero to one risk factor (or above ages and no other risk factors)	<160

Important to our New Rules strategy to outlive heart disease is that these LDL goal levels are only one of the factors that are very significant in determining your risk. Each of the three types of cholesterol should be brought to ideal levels when possible. For most of us a good rule of thumb is an LDL of 130mg/dl or less unless we have a history of coronary heart disease (a heart attack, angina, a bypass operation, angioplasty, or a positive stress test or other noninvasive test) or are diabetic, in which case the LDL cholesterol should be below 70mg. Achieving such a low LDL level will, in most cases, necessitate drug therapy and a change in our diet, details of which will be discussed in subsequent chapters.

OTHER IMPORTANT RISK FACTORS

Cholesterol levels in the blood are important, but so are other risk factors for developing heart disease, as described below.

Blood Pressure (BP)

High blood pressure, also called hypertension, is an increase above a healthy level of the pressure of the blood in our arteries. This is a major treatable cause of heart attacks and strokes. An easy way to understand the numbers (for example, 120/80) used to report this pressure is to think of the left ventricle of the heart contracting with each beat and ejecting blood into the aorta and its branching arteries. This sudden infusion of blood forces the artery to expand to accept it, and the resistance to this expansion by the somewhat elastic wall of the artery will generate a rise in pressure. This highest pressure achieved, usually at the peak of the ejection of blood, is called the systolic pressure and is ideally at or below 120mmHg. With the end of the ejection of blood by the heart, blood in our arteries runs off into the distal blood vessels that supply our organs, and the pressure in the artery falls. The lowest pressure in the artery, before the next heart beat, is the bottom number, ideally 80mmHg or below, and is termed the diastolic blood pressure.

> The units of blood pressure are millimeters of mercury; 120 millimeters of mercury is the pressure required to hold up a column of mercury that is 120 millimeters high (for reference, 1 inch is approximately 25 millimeters). Older machines to measure blood pressure actually used glass tubes marked with a scale in millimeters on the sides filled with mercury. (The danger of mercury to the environment has moved us to use a different type of measuring device.)

The Framingham data demonstrate a clear relationship of elevated blood pressure to heart attacks and cardiovascular death as well as to strokes, heart failure, and kidney failure. Elevation of the systolic (top) pressure is as important a risk as the diastolic (bottom) number. When several large trials were looked at together, it was found that for every 20mmHg increase in the systolic blood pressure or 10mmHg increase in the diastolic blood pressure, cardiovascular risk doubles!

The Joint National Committee (JNC) on prevention, evaluation, and treatment is an NCEP ATP–like group that updates guidelines for determining and treating high blood pressure. The most recent report (2003) breaks downs blood pressure as follows:

Classification	Systolic BP	Diastolic BP
Normal	<120	<80
Pre-hypertension	120–139	80–90
Stage 1 Hypertension	140–159	90–99
Stage 2 Hypertension	>160	>100

For most of us this means that a blood pressure above 120/80 and below 140/90 signals that we should modify our diet and exercise regularly and have our blood pressure checked twice a year. For a blood pressure greater than 140/90 (when either systolic or diastolic pressure is higher than the upper range of pre-hypertension), medication should be prescribed, in addition to making diet modifications and often increasing the frequency and intensity with which we exercise.

Medications are extremely effective in controlling high blood pressure. One medication or a combination of medications that are effective and free of side effects can almost always be found by working with your doctor.

The most commonly used medications to reduce blood pressure include:

- Diuretics (water pills)
- Beta-blocking drugs (which inhibit the effect of your own adrenalin on your heart and blood vessels)
- Calcium channel-blocking drugs (which relax the muscles around your arteries so that they expand, allowing your blood pressure to fall)
- Angiotensin-converting enzymes and their cousin, angiotensin-receptor blockers (which diminish the adrenalin-like effect of a substance in our body called angiotensin II)

Other less commonly used and more potent drugs actually work in the brain to reduce the impulses that elevate blood pressure.

What is important here is the knowledge that for almost all of us, as we age we will develop high blood pressure, truly a "silent killer" because we don't usually feel its effects on a daily basis. Women in particular tend to have lower blood pressure readings than comparably aged men in early life, but women's pressure rises after menopause and must be checked regularly after age 50. African Americans tend to have higher blood pressure readings than Caucasians of the same age. Therefore, an important New Rule to outlive heart disease is to have our blood pressure checked at least each year and to work with our doctors to arrive at a drug or combination of drugs, if needed, that lowers our blood pressure without disturbing side effects. But, *most important* is to take our prescribed medication every day! Remembering to take our blood pressure medications will add good and productive years to our lives.

One-half of all women by the age of 65 will have developed high blood pressure. This is a greater concern for African American women, for whom the risk and prevalence of high blood pressure is greater than for white women. Stroke, which along with cardiac disease is causally related to high blood pressure, is of special concern to women, in whom it is the second-leading cause of cardiovascular mortality. Over 100,000 women die of stroke each year, and many more survive with disability. Of particular concern is the incidence of stroke in African American women. It is almost twice that of Caucasian women!

One current development that is New Rule–worthy is the value of blood pressure readings taken at home by a family member or by ourselves, using home blood pressure measuring devices. The newer generation of these devices is very simple to use, requiring only that we place the device on our arm or forearm, press a button, and write down the readings we see on a digital screen. Blood pressure as measured by these devices correlates as well or better with your heart or stroke risk as the reading taken in your doctor's office, once the doctor has checked to see that the two devices get the same (or nearly the same) readings. The newest American Heart Association guidelines call for doctors to consider treating blood pressure that is high on home blood pressure measurement, even if the level is lower in the office! I suggest to all my patients with elevated or borderline elevated blood pressure (pre-hypertension) that they consider using such a device. Also, since the majority of people will have elevated blood pressure and will lower their cardiac and stroke risk after age 70 with drug therapy, it is a good idea for people with normal blood pressure in their 60s to buy, doctor-check, and use a home device on a monthly basis. Two elevated readings taken at home are a good reason to see your doctor.

> Be especially vigilant about detecting and treating high blood pressure if you are African American or have close family members (parents, brothers or sisters, or children) with high blood pressure.

Smoking Cigarettes/Passive Smoking

Cigarette smoking is perhaps the most preventable cause of coronary heart disease. The Framingham data show that men who smoke have up to 10 times the likelihood of sudden death as nonsmokers and that women smokers have 4.5 times the risk of sudden death. The Nurses Health Study reported even more alarming data, stating that women who smoke a pack or more of cigarettes a day have a fivefold increase in the risk of coronary disease and heart attack when compared to nonsmoking women. Men and women both have an increase in cholesterol and triglyceride readings compared to nonsmokers, and smokers of both genders are more insulin resistant and oxidize more LDL cholesterol than nonsmokers, but *the increase in heart attack risk is greater, per cigarette smoked, in women* than in men!

The "culprit" chemicals in cigarette smoke are most probably nicotine and carbon monoxide. The precise mechanisms that promote atherosclerosis and plaque instability are not well defined, but a myriad of effects that promote atherosclerosis are noted in people who smoke, including constriction of blood vessels; increased platelet "stickiness," which causes an enhancement of the blood clotting mechanism; and a reduction in the blood's oxygen-carrying capacity. Also, inhaled cigarette smoke will cause dysfunction of the smoker's endothelial cells, a clear and probable linkage to atherosclerosis and heart attacks.

As is the case with every poison, the damage cigarette smoke causes is related to the dosage. The longer a person smokes and the number of cigarettes he or she smokes are factors in dosage. The duration factor is noted in the relative risk of heart attacks, which is increased in younger individuals but doubles that of nonsmokers by ages 40 to 50. Even smoking four cigarettes a day or fewer was noted to double relative risk of heart attack in the Coronary Artery Surgery Study in the United States. According to this study, quitting wins a gold star in beating heart disease! Quitters had *one-half* the likelihood of having a second heart attack as people who continued to smoke.

The effect of passive smoking—inhaling smoke from another person's cigarette—has been studied and the surprisingly negative impact on cardiovascular health is the basis for legislation banning indoor smoking in the workplace and in restaurants and bars. A large study (32,000 subjects) of the effect of passive smoking on women was published in 1997 in the medical journal *Circulation*, the official journal of the American Heart Association. The data revealed that women exposed to repeated passive smoke on the job or at home (that is, they lived with a partner who smoked) almost doubled their risk of heart attack. One study also found endothelial cell dysfunction in patients exposed to passive smoke. Of greatest concern is the report in the *Journal of the American Medical Association (JAMA)*, published in 2005, from a large study of atherosclerosis and risk factors that used ultrasound to noninvasively measure the degree of thickening of the inner layer of the carotid artery in an individual. Subjects who reported exposure to passive smoke had 20 percent greater thickening than did those who had not reported smoke exposure. These are *long lasting and probably permanent* changes in the wall of the artery that reflect the pathology behind the increased heart attack rate in people exposed to passive smoke.

The rule is simple: *Try everything* you can to stop smoking if you are a smoker (some more about this later) and *avoid* working or living with people who do smoke. Often, avoiding cigarette smoke is not easy, since advocating for a no-smoking workplace or enforcing an existing policy will not make you popular with addicted smokers at the job (although the rest of your colleagues will likely appreciate your efforts), and will certainly be a source of stress at home. Remember, however, that having your partner give up smoking is a "heartfelt gift" for both of you!

The critical issue in stopping smoking is not "Should I do it?" but rather "How do I do it?" If there were an easy method to stop, one in four Americans would not continue to smoke.

You can succeed with a will to try *repeatedly*, since the average successful ex-smoker (defined as someone who has not smoked in one year) will have tried eight times prior to his or her successful attempt.

Specific counseling from a physician has been shown to be a powerful motivating influence in quitting, especially when the doctor or his office staff follows up on how well the patient is doing. At your next appointment, if you are not definitively told to stop smoking, ask the physician about your smoking, how dangerous it is, and how much healthier you will be and how much better you will feel when you stop. Doctors have been found to more often counsel men than women, whites than minority patients, and heavy smokers than light smokers. If your doctor doesn't provide you with adequate information and advice, you can call the various national smoke-ending organizations—or get a different doctor!

> In the Nurses Health Study, women who had stopped smoking had a 30 percent lower risk of heart disease after two years, compared with women who continued to smoke. One important barrier to smoking cessation in women was identified: when cessation was associated with weight gain—and it often initially is—the women returned to smoking. Diet and exercise programs to prevent weight gain can play an important role in smoking cessation in women.

Type II Diabetes

See the discussion of triglycerides, above, and metabolic syndrome, which follows, for a clear picture of the role diabetes plays in the development of atherosclerosis and heart disease.

Diet

The role of diet in raising total and LDL cholesterol is well defined, but it is now clear that the risk or protective value of a diet goes well beyond its effect on blood lipids, blood pressure, and obesity. Studies that compared death rates in different countries noted a large relative reduction in heart attack and heart-event death rates in populations that ate diets rich in fruits, vegetables, grains, and cold-water fish. In the 25-year follow-up to the World Health Organization's Seven Countries Study of heart disease, the heart attack–heart death risk of a person with a cholesterol level of 225mg/dl in northern Europe was much higher than the person with the same cholesterol in a Mediterranean country, a finding not explained by differences in smoking or high blood pressure. Also, clinical trials that assigned patients to a diet similar to that consumed in Mediterranean countries have shown a very impressive reduction in second cardiac events. In the battle against heart disease, we are what we eat—and adjusting our eating patterns to favor specific food types provides a powerful and tasty New Rule strategy! (See New Rule No. 5, beginning on page 96.)

Sedentary Lifestyle

Regular physical activity in the context of work, recreation, or an exercise training program is associated with a marked reduction in heart disease–related death in patients after heart attacks, bypass surgery, or angioplasty. Numerous studies, including the Framingham study, have evaluated populations by how much physical activity they perform and shown that, in almost all cases, the more activity the population performs, the lower is its risk of heart attack. Patients who do not engage in a moderately strenuous activity such as walking, cycling, dancing, or swimming—to name just a few heart-healthy activities—are at significantly increased risk of a heart attack. In addition, patients who have heart disease and then join programs that include exercise and diet modification increase the number of years they live by more than 10 percent. This is an enormously powerful effect and thus the basis of a key New Rules strategy. (See New Rule No. 4, beginning on page 73.)

Metabolic Syndrome

When evaluating your lipid profile after receiving the results of your blood test, ask your doctor whether you have metabolic syndrome. You have this condition if any three of the following five factors apply to you:

- Abdominal obesity (for men, a waist greater than 40 inches; for women, a waist greater than 35 inches)
- Triglycerides greater than 150mg/dl
- Low HDL cholesterol (for men, less than 40mg/dl; for women, less than 50mg/dl)
- Blood pressure over 130/85
- Fasting blood sugar greater than 110mg/dl

This syndrome is now understood to relate to your body's resistance to its own insulin. This resistance means that the insulin-producing cells in your pancreas must produce more insulin to allow your cells to take in enough blood sugar (this is the major function of your insulin). The increased insulin itself circulating in the bloodstream promotes atherosclerosis, and the low HDL and high triglycerides are significant coronary heart disease (CHD) risk factors. If you meet these criteria and if your lipid profile shows a low HDL and high triglycerides, you have metabolic syndrome and are at increased risk of coronary heart disease and of developing diabetes. In addition to your LDL cholesterol levels, your HDL cholesterol and triglycerides are also important targets for therapy, and treatment for all three is now considered imperative in order to reduce risk and outlive heart disease.

Treatment of metabolic syndrome should include a combination of diet, exercise, and drug therapy. Reasonable treatment approaches can include taking a statin, statins plus niacin, or fibric acid drugs (Lopid or Tricor), and in some cases, fish oil capsules. You should monitor the response to the initial therapy and understand your doctor's decision to raise the dose or change drugs on the basis of achieving all three goals:

- Reducing LDL
- Raising HDL
- Reducing triglycerides

If your LDL and triglyceride levels are not reduced on your second blood test and your doctor is not addressing this issue, *ask why!* Although there is not a recommended HDL target treatment goal, I use 45 in men and 55 in women. If, however, the patient can't tolerate niacin, it will not, in some instances, be possible to achieve the HDL goal.

OTHER MAJOR RISK FACTORS (IN ADDITION TO THE FRAMINGHAM STUDY'S FINDINGS)

Depression

Several studies have confirmed the link between depression and risk of coronary events. In fact, the connection is so significant that I devote an entire chapter to the mind-body connection with regard to heart attack risk. See New Rule No. 6 (beginning on page 118).

C-Reactive Protein (CRP)

This protein is produced by your liver when white blood cells involved in an inflammatory process secrete a substance called interlukin-6 (IL6). New techniques allow us to measure CRP more precisely. High CRP levels indicate an active process of inflammation in the walls of the arteries. *CRP levels predict heart attacks with the same accuracy as LDL cholesterol levels.* So for risk assessment, CRP can be an important measurement, especially if your cholesterol places you in an intermediate risk range. Depending on your risk, you should have CRP measured as part of an initial evaluation or as a follow-up blood test. We do not yet have clinical trials showing which treatment strategies work to lower CRP and reduce coronary events. Why? Because this is relatively new science. The goal, then, with an elevated CRP measurement is to reduce overall heart attack risk—by lowering LDL cholesterol with a statin, for instance. Statins are also one of the very few drugs that reduce CRP by means of a yet-unknown mechanism (possibly an anti-inflammatory effect). Stopping cigarette smoking has been associated with a reduction in CRP, as has regular exercise, all part of a global risk reduction program. Until we have studies that prove the effectiveness of a drug for reducing CRP, for now the answer is to do everything else to lower overall heart attack risk and to use a statin if overall risk is high. (See New Rule No. 3, beginning on page 58.)

Homocysteine

For some time doctors have known that children born with a rare genetic condition known as homocysteinuria, which produces high blood levels of an amino acid called homocysteine, developed severe atherosclerosis at a very young age. Recently we have learned that almost 10 percent of us are born with a gene that causes a slight increase in our serum homocysteine, which is associated with an increased risk of atherosclerosis and heart attacks. The pathway responsible for the prompt removal of homocysteine from our blood depends on specific enzymes that are less active in people born with the tendency to have higher-than-normal homocysteine. Luckily, the enzymes can be stimulated to work at a more normal pace by ingesting higher amounts of certain B vitamins, specifically folic acid, with smaller amounts of B6 and B12. This vitamin regimen will reduce homocysteine, but a large recent study showed no protective effect and in some instances an increase in the risk of heart attack and stroke.

Lp(a)

The Lp(a) particle has two distinct parts. One part looks like LDL cholesterol and the other looks like a substance in our blood that helps dissolve early clots called plasmin. The data indicates that Lp(a), when elevated, may both promote atherosclerosis by its LDL cholesterol part, *and* interfere with our normal ability to dissolve clots by the plasmin-looking particles, a kind of double whammy. Our levels are genetically determined, with levels over 30mg/dl considered abnormal. Only high doses of niacin have been shown to lower Lp(a), and niacin does so only modestly. But niacin in high doses has unpleasant side effects—flushing and gastrointestinal difficulties—in almost half of my patients. Therefore, when these values are high, the current treatment strategy is to get your LDL cholesterol to low-target ranges and address all other risk factors to lower your total risk.

HOW TO SCORE YOUR 10-YEAR RISK OF HAVING A HEART ATTACK

The purpose of this chapter is to provide enough information to allow you to estimate your risk of having a heart attack in the next 10 years and prompt you to have a conversation with your doctor about appropriate testing and medications if your risk is in the moderate or high ranges. You can use the NCEP ATP Framingham risk scoring pages to help assess your individual risk. The scoring pages follow.

ESTIMATE OF 10-YEAR RISK FOR MEN
(Framingham Point Scores)

Age Chart	Points
20–34	-9
35–39	-4
40–44	0
45–49	3
50–54	6
55–59	8
60–64	10
65–69	11
70–74	12
75–79	13

Total Cholesterol Chart	Points at ages 20–39	Points at ages 40–49	Points at ages 50–59	Points at ages 60–69	Points at ages 70–79
<160	0	0	0	0	0
160–199	4	3	2	1	0
200–239	7	5	3	1	0
240–270	9	6	4	2	1
≥280	11	8	5	3	1
NONSMOKER	0	0	0	0	0
SMOKER	8	5	3	1	1

MEN HDL CHART

HDL	POINTS
≥60	-1
50–59	0
40–49	1
<40	2

MEN BP CHART

Systolic BP	If Untreated	If Treated
<120	0	0
120–129	0	1
130–139	1	2
140–159	1	2
>160	2	3

FRAMINGHAM MEN POINT TOTAL SCORES

Point Total	10-Year Risk %
<0	<1
0	1
1	1
2	1
3	1
4	1
5	2
6	2
7	3
8	4
9	5
10	6
11	8
12	10
13	12
14	16
15	20
16	25
$\geq$17	$\geq$30

ESTIMATE OF 10-YEAR RISK FOR WOMEN
(Framingham Point Scores)

Age Chart	Points
20–34	-7
35–39	-3
40–44	0
45–49	3
50–54	6
55–59	8
60–64	10
65–69	12
70–74	14
75–79	16

Total Cholesterol Chart	Points at ages 20–39	Points at ages 40–49	Points at ages 50–59	Points at ages 60–69	Points at ages 70–79
<160	0	0	0	0	0
160–199	4	3	2	1	1
200–239	8	6	4	2	1
240–270	11	8	5	3	2
≥280	13	10	7	4	2
NONSMOKER	0	0	0	0	0
SMOKER	9	7	4	2	1

WOMEN HDL CHART

HDL	POINTS
≥60	-1
50–59	0
40–49	1
<40	2

WOMEN BP CHART

Systolic BP	If Untreated	If Treated
<1200	0	
120–129	1	3
130–139	2	4
140–159	3	5
≥160	4	6

FRAMINGHAM WOMEN POINT TOTAL SCORES

Point Total	10-Year Risk %
<9	<1
9	1
10	1
11	1
12	1
13	2
14	2
15	3
16	4
17	5
18	6
19	8
20	11
21	14
22	17
23	22
24	27
>25	>30

Here's what you need to know to use the pages and make them a document useful to your physician. I'll use myself as an example for how you should approach this questionnaire.

The NCEP ATP Framingham risk scoring page I'll use is for men; women have a different page with different information. Let's walk through this together, using my numbers and history. Then you should do yours!

First, look at the **Age Chart** and circle the number associated with your age. Using the male gender page, I give myself 10 points for being in the 60- to 64-year-old range.

Next, look at the **Total Cholesterol Chart**. I give myself 1 point for my age (65) and a total cholesterol between 160 and 199.

Next, look at the **HDL Chart**. I give myself 1 for an HDL between 40 and 49.

Next, look at the **Systolic Blood Pressure (BP) Chart**. I get zero points for a systolic blood pressure (without treatment) of less than 129.

Next, look at the **Smoking Chart**. I get zero for being a nonsmoker.

My total point value is 13 and, when I locate that number on the **Risk Chart**, I note that my 10-year risk of a heart event is 12 percent, a number that puts me in the "intermediate (6 to 20 percent) risk" range. This is the range in which a CRP measurement can be of value, since, if it is high, it might increase my risk to the "high (over 20 percent)" range. In fact, I know my value and it puts me solidly in the intermediate range. In consultation with my doctor, I chose to have an exercise EKG nuclear examination at a nuclear imaging lab (the one I established at Downstate Medical School). On the basis of a "very good" exercise duration and the absence of exercise-induced symptoms, and EKG changes or abnormalities on the nuclear isotope scans, my physician and I concurred that further testing is not indicated, but that continued aggressive New Rules prevention and awareness is!

If my exercise nuclear examination had been significantly positive, meaning I had chest pain or changes on my EKG or a defect on my nuclear scan, the results would have indicated an increased likelihood of a significantly narrowed artery and the possibility of coronary atherosclerosis. Depending on how much disease was seen, I might then have undergone a coronary angiogram to rule out the kind of extensive disease that would be an indication for an angioplasty procedure or coronary artery bypass surgery. I am thankful I did not need such a procedure, but if the testing and the angiogram had indicated the type of disease in which outcome is very much improved with angioplasty or surgery, I would have been thankful that I had the testing performed.

YOUR 10-YEAR RISK: DETERMINING WHAT TO DO NEXT

The key here is what to do once you have calculated your risk. The appropriate responses are as follows.

> Remember that this plan assumes the absence of a prior heart attack or diagnosis of coronary artery disease as well as the absence of "associated disease" (such as diabetes) or important symptoms. *In these instances aggressive treatment and often further testing are needed, even if your Framingham risk score is low.*

Remember: Low Risk Is NOT No Risk!

About 5 percent of the population with a low-risk score will have a heart attack within 10 years. Therefore, you need to be aware of other risk factors and address increased levels with a New Rules–type heart-healthy diet and exercise program and, when appropriate, medications.

Also,

- Have all age-appropriate screening evaluations.
- Recognize and respond to depression.
- Be alert to the onset of symptoms (see New Rule No. 1, beginning on page 17) that might signal that heart disease is developing.

Remember: you want to do everything you can to avoid being one of the 5 percent or so of low-risk patients who will have a heart attack over the next 10 years.

Intermediate Risk: Become Vigilant about Your Heart Health!

- Look with your doctor at other risk factors that might move you up even further in risk, such as an elevated CRP or Lp(a) level.
- Discuss your status with regard to symptoms and associated diseases (such as diabetes and obesity) with your doctor. Address the issues of further cardiac testing and if so, which ones.
- Aggressively reduce risk factors (major and minor) with diet, exercise, and medications, if appropriate, and look at your responses to the questions in the mind-body

chapter (New Rule No. 6, beginning on page 118). If more than one or two are answered in the affirmative, consider one or more of the programs suggested in that chapter.

Lowering your intermediate risk to as close to optimal levels as possible; taking part in a proactive exercise and diet program; addressing psychosocial factors such as depression, hostility, anxiety, and social support; and maintaining an open vigilant awareness of symptoms that may indicate the presence of heart disease are critical factors to outliving heart disease. Discuss with your doctor whether you need further testing and the specific test you might need, and make sure you have careful follow-up evaluations. These steps are essential components to a program that will optimize your chances of outliving heart disease.

High Risk: Consider This Information Your Wake-up Call!

In this category you have a *greater than* 1-in-5 chance of a cardiac event over the next 10 years. This is important information and a wake-up call to do everything possible to prevent or outlive the event. Your strategy should include:

- A comprehensive risk-assessment and risk-reduction analysis
- Assessment of your current cardiovascular status using tests such as nuclear stress imaging and appropriate follow-up studies

A comprehensive New Rules approach to strategies will help keep you out of the 20 percent event-rate group. The subsequent chapters of this book will provide you with the information and guidelines to maximize your chances of doing exactly that.

Evaluating your risk of having a heart attack or developing heart disease critical enough to warrant treatment to prevent heart attack is essential to outliving your heart disease. The next chapter offers information about a treatment to prevent heart attack so effective that even doctors and medical researchers consider it is almost too good to be true.

TAKE A STATIN IF YOU NEED IT! THESE MIRACLE DRUGS (AND OTHER IMPORTANT DRUGS FOR DYSLIPIDEMIA) HAVE A HUGE ROLE IN MAINTAINING HEART HEALTH

Statins and the other powerful drugs that improve our cholesterol levels are so important that they deserve a top spot in our discussion of the New Rules to outlive heart disease. You probably know the old adage, "if something seems too good to be true, it probably is" (too good to be true). If someone tries to sell you the Brooklyn Bridge, that's a good adage to keep in mind. But statins and related drugs are the exception; they work very effectively not only to block the production of the kind of cholesterol that can turn our blood vessels into pockets of plaque, but also to stop the process that leads these plaques to fracture and cause a heart attack. This chapter explains how we discovered their effectiveness and why they are truly miracle drugs in combating heart disease. It also looks at the drug's limitations and the newer approaches to drug therapy that are being developed.

THE GOOD NEWS ABOUT STATINS

Early clinical scientists observed that atherosclerotic plaques were composed in large part of cholesterol deposits in their center, and many international studies confirmed that populations with elevated cholesterol in the blood had an increased risk of coronary heart disease. The initial findings from the Framingham study showed that the greater the cholesterol levels in the blood, the higher the risk of developing heart disease, and that this risk increased when other factors, such as high blood pressure and smoking, were part of a person's profile. The critical piece of evidence showing that reducing LDL cholesterol would reduce atherosclerosis and heart attacks was difficult to obtain, since the early cholesterol-lowering drugs were a class of chemicals called resins, which work by binding to the liver's bile acids and preventing their normal absorption by the intestines. The loss of these resin-bound bile acids in our stool forces the body to use cholesterol circulating in the bloodstream to make new bile acids. Resins worked to lower cholesterol, but only modestly. Before the introduction of statins, the very low-fat diets were a way to lower cholesterol levels, but these controlled eating plans were so restrictive that patients found them difficult to adhere to.

The introduction of lovastatin (Mevacor), the first of a class of drugs called statins, overcame these barriers—statins proved very effective and were easy to take. Statins were developed to work differently from resins. Rather than bind to bile acids, they were developed to inhibit a liver enzyme (acetyl co-A reductace) from performing a critical step in the synthesis of LDL cholesterol. The LDL cholesterol never forms and therefore cannot be circulated in the blood. Statins allowed physicians, for the first time, to reduce a patient's LDL cholesterol by up to 50 percent, to low-risk levels, in the overwhelming majority of patients. Statins also have a low incidence of side effects and drug reactions. The pharmaceutical and medical communities saw statins as having the potential to "regress" atherosclerosis, that is, to turn back the atherosclerotic clock and return a patient's arteries to a much lower level of disease, with fewer and smaller obstructing atherosclerotic plaques.

With this "dream" and the potential financial implications of achieving actual plaque regression in mind, a series of studies were funded by drug companies and performed by academic clinical scientists. One of these studies was called the Familiar Atherosclerosis Treatment Study, otherwise known as FATS, published in 1990. The FATS researchers recruited patients with coronary heart disease who had had a recent angiogram as part of their treatment. These were controlled studies, meaning that one group of patients, assigned at random, received the statin and, in some cases, a statin plus another medication, and the other group received a placebo, or so-called sugar pill, instead of a statin.

Because statins have been shown to be so effective, it would now be unethical to withhold statin treatment from any patient. Before the FATS and other similar studies, there was no convincing clinical evidence that lowering cholesterol with statins would change clinical outcome and so it was ethical to treat a group of patients with placebo.

After one year, the two groups had blood tests to remeasure their lipid levels and were again given angiograms to measure the amount of coronary artery atherosclerosis. The two angiograms of each patient were compared.

Scientists found that the statin drugs significantly lowered the LDL cholesterol levels, but they did *not* find a reduction in the number or size of the plaques, which is what they expected to see. They were disappointed that there was not more "improvement" in the before and after angiograms. There was some evidence that more plaques regressed and fewer enlarged in the statin patients than in the placebo patients, but only in the 2 to 4 percent range, an unimpressive statistic because the differences in scoring the angiograms, despite computer-assisted techniques, differed among skilled observers by as much as 5 percent!

But far more impressive were the differences in clinical outcome of the patients in the statin and placebo groups. Even though the angiograms did not dramatically change in the one-year test period, the incidence of heart attacks, sudden cardiac death, and admission to a hospital for bypass surgery dropped in the statin patients by a full one-third. This finding was consistently seen in study after study of patients and controls who were also being treated for other risk factors, such as high blood pressure, and counseled to exercise and stop smoking. In another part of the FATS study, a small group of patients was selected randomly to receive lovastatin (Mevacor) and the vitamin niacin (to lower LDL and to raise HDL). Compared to a group receiving a placebo, the treatment group had more than two-thirds reduction in clinical events!

These results changed the rules for winning the battle against heart disease. Despite minimal improvement in the size of the plaques in the angiograms, the statin-treated patients were having far fewer heart attacks and living longer. What followed were a series of studies with lovastatin (Mevacor) and other drugs—such as pravastatin (Pravachol); simvastatin (Zocor); and, most recently, atorvastatin (Lipitor)—to study the clinical outcomes in patients with heart disease.

A large study in Sweden—the Scandinavian Simvastatin Survival (or 4S) study—of 4,444 people who had heart disease and were randomly placed on simvastatin (Zocor) or placebo, was conceived in 1987 and reported at the seven-year mark in the British medical journal *The Lancet* (November 19, 1994). This

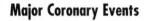

Major Coronary Events

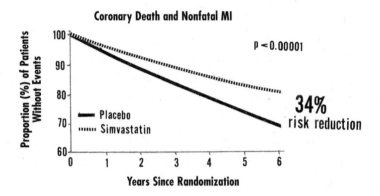

study focused on clinical outcome of heart patients from four Scandanavian countries (Sweden, Finland, Norway, and Denmark); angiograms were not part of the study. In other words, the researchers wanted to know whether patients taking simvastatin (Zocor) have fewer heart attacks and other significant heart problems than a control group.

This study revealed a 34 percent reduction in heart attack deaths in the patients who took the statin as compared to the group who took a placebo. Several important pieces of clinically important information were produced by this study.

- One was the finding that the reduction in death from heart attacks was as true for women with heart disease as for men (earlier studies had not enrolled enough women to reach this conclusion).
- Another was the finding of the reduction of clinical events in patients with diabetes.
- Of equal importance was the finding that symptoms that could be considered drug complications, such as

headache, nausea, fatigue, joint or muscle pain, were not significantly different during the seven-year period between those taking the drug and those on the placebo.

Statins do have side effects that in some cases require the patient to stop taking them, and in very rare instances these side effects are serious enough to be life threatening. The overwhelming majority of us, however, will experience no side effects.

Three other major studies are worth noting, since they form the foundation of the New Rule regarding the treatment of dyslipidemia (high cholesterol). The West of Scotland Coronary Prevention Study, known as WOSCOP and performed, of course, in the western region of Scotland, enrolled men with increased cholesterol levels but who did not have heart disease. The men were placed either on a statin (in this study, pravastatin) or placebo. The five-year follow-up, reported in 1995, showed that first heart attacks and other cardiac events were significantly reduced in the men who took the statin. This study showed clearly that the statins are effective at protecting men at increased risk of developing heart disease as well as those who have already developed it. The Air Force–Texas Coronary Artery Prevention Project, reported in 2003, enrolled men and women with moderate elevations in cholesterol, a profile that fits nearly one-third of the adults in the United States. The statin group was treated with lovastatin (Mevacor) and, again, showed a significant reduction in first heart attacks. Finally, the Atorvastatin Versus Revascularization Treatments (commonly referred to as the AVERT trial), reported in 2004, enrolled patients with angina pectoris (chest pain) whose angiograms showed a single significant narrowing of one of the three main coronary arteries. Patients were chosen at random to undergo angioplasty with stenting or to take atorvastatin (Lipitor) at a high dose for six months. Clinical outcomes (which measured, for example, worsening symptoms and heart attacks) were slightly better in those who took the statins.

HOW STATINS WORK

How do statins work to reduce coronary events in those with already-formed plaques and atherosclerosis? When these drugs were discovered, we understood that they reduced LDL cholesterol in the blood, but our understanding of just what made heart attacks happen wasn't perfected. Once we understood the difference between stable plaques and unstable ones in the role of heart attacks, we began to understand that the statins, in addition to lowering cholesterol, actually make the plaques that already existed more stable and less likely to fracture. The hope was that the lower cholesterol levels would, in essence, turn back the clock and give us the blood vessels of 20-year-olds. That didn't happen, but what did result were plaques that were less likely to get inflamed and fracture. With less risk of fracture, patients did not develop the clots that can result in a heart attack.

The statins work in a variety of ways. They primarily work by reducing the amount of LDL cholesterol in our blood, so that less LDL cholesterol crosses into our artery walls and therefore fewer plaques are formed.

We are just beginning to understand that statins may have a second and very important role: We call these the plieotropic (other) effects of statins, the things these drugs do beyond the main job. The other direct effect of statins may be to decrease the process of oxidation, which triggers the inflammatory response, and thereby limit LDL cholesterol damage to arteries. In other words, statins may directly reduce, or inhibit, inflammation that leads to plaque rupture in the blood vessels.

How did we become aware of a possible secondary effect? Statins act very quickly to reduce the number of heart attacks in those taking the medication, more quickly than can be explained by simply lowering LDL cholesterol. If the only effect of statins was to lower cholesterol, it would take a long time to see a reduction in heart attack rate among those taking the drug. Since the rate comes down dramatically and quickly, there must be a secondary reason for statins' effectiveness.

Statins have become dramatically important drugs. Initially we used them to treat people with high cholesterol, and then we started lowering the level of what we considered to be "normal" cholesterol levels in patients with heart disease. We learned that if we thought an LDL level of 160ml/db was high, we could lower it to 130, and now we've learned that after a heart attack, or if a patient has heart disease of any kind, lowering LDL to 60 or 70 with the help of a statin will dramatically reduce the chances of her having a second heart attack. These drugs are extraordinarily powerful.

Most Heart Attacks Are Due to the Rupture of Small Plaques*

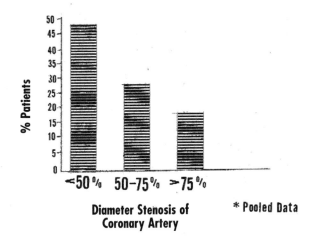

% Patients

Diameter Stenosis of Coronary Artery

<50% 50–75% >75%

* Pooled Data

Side Effects of Statins

Some patients can't take statins because they have experienced negative side effects, such as muscle weakness or pain, or increases in liver or muscle enzymes that indicate a toxic effect on that organ. For these patients or for those for whom drugs that impact on high triglycerides or low HDL as well as LDL cholesterol are a better clinical choice, there is a variety of other powerful cholesterol-lowering drugs that can be prescribed.

Alternatives to statins include:

- Fibric acids (Lopid and Tricor), a class of drugs that work in the liver at a different step in the creation of cholesterol than do statins
- Niacin in doses of 1 to 2 grams a day, which is 20 to 40 times higher than the dose found in vitamin supplements
- Newer forms of the resins that bind to bile acids
- Drugs such as ezetimide (Zetia) that interfere with the cholesterol receptors on the inside wall of the intestines, and, when used with statins, enhance the statins' effects. Patients can then take much lower doses of statins and may be able to achieve the same cholesterol-lowering benefits without the muscle soreness

Although LDL cholesterol is generally lower in premenopausal women than in men, it rises quickly after menopause, so that women in their 60s to 90s will generally have higher LDL cholesterol levels than men. The important take-home message is that women have to increase the frequency of their lipoprotein blood tests after menopause to twice a year, be more assiduous at adopting a heart-healthy diet and exercise program, and take cholesterol-lowering medications if indicated.

New Science and Statins

Three studies have reported the use of high doses of statins to bring cholesterol down to very low levels—60 to 70ml/db with, for the first time, a regression in the size and number of atherosclerotic plaques! (You may remember from the Introduction and the earlier discussion in this chapter that statins prevent heart attacks even without a reduction in the size and number of plaques—plaque regression—that researchers expected to find.) Among this group are studies by Dr. Nissen and colleagues from the Cleveland Clinic, published in the *New England Journal of Medicine*, using a technique called intravascular echocardiography, which creates a picture of the inside walls of the arteries. This is done using sonar that is better than angiograms to measure the extent of atherosclerosis. Using the highest dose of atorvastatin (Lipitor), investigators were able reduce LDL cholesterol to well below 70mg/dl and saw, on the intravascular ultrasound, regression of the plaques. Recall that we could not convincingly see such regression on the doses we were administering a decade ago in the angiography studies. Now, with higher doses of statins and more sensitive ways to measure atherosclerosis, these studies are showing us that we can shrink plaque and turn back the clock for our arteries.

How Low to Go?

As we discussed in the previous chapter, the NCEP APT, which sets guidelines for optimal cholesterol levels based on a person's risk factors for developing heart disease, lowered their recommended levels in 2004. The question that now intrigues researchers is how low those cholesterol levels should go.

Scientists have noted that most people living a contemporary lifestyle have an average total cholesterol of 220, with an LDL of about 130. But this average cholesterol level is associated with an unacceptable risk of atherosclerosis development, heart attacks, and death. We now treat to LDL levels of 70mg/dl in patients with heart disease. Is there a case to be made for lowering LDL cholesterol levels in all adults to 70mg/dl and to 50mg/dl in patients with atherosclerotic disease? Could we completely stop the disease's progress at that low a level of LDL cholesterol?

Clinical researchers have used two very different types of information to address this question. Various studies showed that the lower we drove cholesterol with higher doses of statins, the lower were the cardiac-event rates, suggesting that there is a dose-response effect (similar to the exercise–heart disease response discussed in the next New Rules chapter on exercise). This would support the concept that the lower you bring down your LDL cholesterol, the greater you would reduce your risk. Researchers then looked at cholesterol levels in the few remaining "primitive" populations (including selected populations of native Eskimo Inuit and Australian pygmies) that continue to live as hunter-gatherers, meaning that they grow, gather, and hunt their food rather than shop for it in a grocery store. These groups have LDL cholesterol levels between 50 and 60 and only very rarely have heart disease. The researchers also looked at our nearest animal cousins—chimpanzees and apes—and noted that they almost all have LDL cholesterol levels between 50 and 70.

Researchers have theorized that before we developed animal husbandry and civilization, humans had cholesterol levels in the range that chimps, apes, and hunter-gatherers have today. And we had essentially NO heart disease. So, in today's world, is it possible to live with cholesterol levels at that level? The answer is probably not, because we eat prepared foods and very few of us do the physical work that these groups do every day. Researchers then posited that since we now have the ability with these new drugs to safely reduce our LDL levels to those of the hunter-gatherer, might such low cholesterol levels be, in the future, an endorsed clinical goal? Their question is interesting, and deserves further study. Stay tuned!

Too Good to Be True?

Statins are almost too good to be true—except that the clinical results we've noted over the last 20 years are simply undeniable. You should be taking them, or the other powerful drugs to lower high cholesterol levels, if you have coronary heart disease. You should in many cases take them even if you have no heart disease but have high cholesterol levels that have not been brought down by a diet and exercise program. However, you must be aware of two limitations of this rule.

First, keep in mind the side effects of statins, discussed earlier in this chapter. Published data and my clinical experience are that about one in forty patients will have muscle pain; for this reason I will stop the statins, especially if there is an increase in certain blood enzymes that show that the muscles are being affected. In a smaller number of patients, I will stop the statins because of elevations in liver enzymes. Your doctor should do liver enzyme blood testing before starting you on the statins and repeat these tests at one month and again at three months. If there are no abnormalities at this point, I repeat these tests only when I have to increase the dose of the statin or change the specific statin. In addition, the very rare patient (one in between 1 million and 1.5 million) will have a life-threatening complication called rhabdomyolisis, in which muscle cells die rapidly and release proteins into the blood that cause almost immediate kidney failure. Again, this side effect is rare, but it occurs more commonly when the patient requires the combination of a statin and a fibric acid drug.

Second, regarding the studies I refer to on the efficacy of

statins: the facts are that we have studies of sufficient size to show that statins reduce heart attack risk and death in *white men* who already have heart disease (this is called secondary prevention) and in *white men* who do not have clinical signs or evidence of heart disease but have increased risk and elevated cholesterol (this is termed primary prevention). And for *white women*, we have studies that show the value of statins in secondary prevention (that is, the subjects already have heart disease). There are no large studies that have addressed primary prevention in women, in other words, the ability of statins to prevent first heart attacks in women. Doctors prescribe statins for this use in women since, in almost all instances, strategies that work for secondary prevention have worked for primary prevention, and the very large and long-term studies to document the value of statins in primary prevention in women are not yet being done. It seems prudent on the part of doctors to use statins for primary prevention in women, and the NCEP ATP protocols call for such usage.

This same caution applies to African Americans. We do not have sufficiently large numbers in trials to document the presumed value of statins to this group, although doctors think it is prudent to prescribe them when indicated by current guidelines.

THE FUTURE OF DRUG THERAPY IN TREATING HEART DISEASE

What lies ahead in the treatment and prevention of atherosclerosis? Rather than lowering high levels of "bad" cholesterol, scientists are working on drugs that will raise low levels of "good" cholesterol. Additionally, a protein called apoprotein A that is on the surface of the HDL cholesterol particle is the subject of a promising study. One approach to raising HDL cholesterol to lower heart attack risk has focused on drugs that inhibit the activity of a protein in our bodies called CETP that works to lower our HDL. Based on studies showing that people born with genes that produce less CETP had lower risks of heart attack, and on studies in animals and one pilot study in humans, a drug to inhibit CETP was thought to be very promising. Unfortunately, when the full-scale clinical trial was under way, it became clear that the patients randomized to the new drug were not reducing the atherosclerotic plaque in their arteries and had, in fact, a higher incidence of heart events than did the patients randomized to the placebo. The question that remains unanswered is whether the problem is with the concept of inhibiting our CETP to raise HDL or with the specific drug that was being investigated. Time and further scientific developments will, I hope, yield the answer.

Another study is based on the finding over 20 years ago of a population of people with very low HDL but a genetically

---

BENEFITS OF STATINS

- Safe
- Effective
- Inhibit a liver enzyme responsible for LDL synthesis
- Reduce LDL ("bad") cholesterol up to 50 percent
- Reduce inflammation, thus decreasing LDL damage to arteries
- Low incidence of side effects (about 5 percent muscle pain and abnormal liver blood tests); very rare but very toxic rhabdomyolysis
- *In men,* work to reduce first heart attacks
- *In men and women* with heart disease, have been shown to reduce subsequent heart attacks and increase longevity

unique form of a protein, called apoA1Milano, that is attached to HDL cholesterol. This genetically unique protein can now be created in the laboratory and is available as a solution that can be given intravenously. In a small trial of weekly intravenous infusions of this product, people with disease in the coronary arteries had an impressive regression of their plaques when their blood vessels were measured by ultrasound. This treatment is still very experimental and not yet available—but the studies to determine its full effect and safety are starting—and it may be a glimpse of a very bright future in our efforts to outlive heart disease!

EXERCISE! IT'S A PROACTIVE WAY TO REDUCE HEART DISEASE AND HEART ATTACK RISK

Regular exercise is essential to your strategy to outlive heart disease, both before you develop symptoms and after. What's the best exercise program to outlive heart disease? As I explain later in this chapter, the best exercise program for your heart is the one you will stick with. Understanding why exercise is so important to your heart's health may inspire you to do just that.

This chapter begins with a short explanation of what happens to our bodies during exercise and then gives general guidelines about the kind of exercise program you might want to set up and how to perform your workout sessions to provide maximum benefits to your heart.

THE VALUE OF REGULAR EXERCISE

The realization that regular exercise was more than just part of a healthy lifestyle—that it has a powerful impact on a person's chance of developing heart disease—started with the observation in the early 1950s that bus drivers in the city of London had a much higher rate of cardiac-related death than did the conductors, who walked and climbed the double-decker buses as part of their job. Although the correlation was later questioned, the information nevertheless stimulated a series of well-designed studies that defined the relationship between daily physical activity and heart health.

In the mid-1970s Dr. Paffenbarger at the Stanford University School of Medicine initiated a study of the relationship of physical work to the heart disease and death rate of San Francisco dock workers. This study was done before the advent of container shipping, at a time when dock workers who unloaded ships performed heavy manual labor; supervisors, light labor; and office personnel, very light physical activity. The study, after accounting for the risk associated with smoking, high blood pressure, and blood cholesterol level, found that the heavy manual labor dock workers had a much lower cardiac death rate than their lighter-labor coworkers, and that there was no real difference in cardiac disease between the light (walking the docks with a clipboard) and the very light (desk jobs) workers.

A second study performed a decade later, and led by Dr. Paffenbarger, addressed the cardiac-event rate of Harvard College alumni in relation to the physical activity performed while at college and years later, as analyzed from an extensive questionnaire. Harvard's uniquely complete and extensive information files for its alumni, and the high rate of participation in Harvard-sponsored projects by its alumni, made this study possible. The study of almost 17,000 men demonstrated an unequivocal correlation between exercise and reduced heart attack and cardiac death rates, even after accounting for other cardiac risk factors.

The study, however, went beyond finding that regular exercise reduced the risk of heart attack. Two findings are worth mentioning.

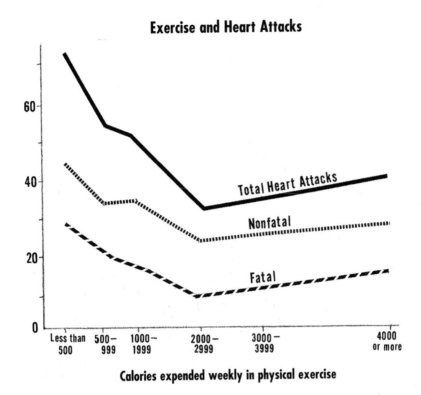

Exercise and Heart Attacks

Total Heart Attacks

Nonfatal

Fatal

Less than 500 | 500–999 | 1000–1999 | 2000–2999 | 3000–3999 | 4000 or more

60
40
20
0

Calories expended weekly in physical exercise

First, the Harvard Alumni study demonstrated a direct relationship between the amount of exercise performed and the likelihood of a cardiac event. This is called a dose-response relationship and is an extraordinarily powerful statistical finding linking weekly exercise with the incidence of cardiac events. Men who expended 3,000 calories or more during their workouts every week had the lowest incidence of heart disease. The average person burns 100 calories walking or running a mile, so these men were performing exercise that was the equivalent of running 30 miles a week. But even by burning 500 to 1,000 calories a week (Kcal/wk), heart-event rates were substantially reduced when compared with the sedentary alumni. The conclusion is that more is better! The single exception, not relevant to most people, was their finding that the group who exceeded 4,000Kcal/wk had a very low, but a slightly higher event rate, than those at 3,000Kcal/wk.

Second, the Harvard Alumni study demonstrated that the amount of exercise a person performed would reduce his heart attack rate independent of the extent of other coronary heart disease risk factors. For example, if you smoked three packs of cigarettes a day, vigorous and regular exercise would reduce risk of a heart attack to a level less than that of the one-pack-a-day smoker. If a person's total cholesterol was very high, regular exercise could reduce the rate of heart attack to that of a person with a modest elevation. And the more exercise a person performed, the lower the cardiac-event rate.

One study that addressed the short- and long-term cardio-protective value of engaging in regular exercise activities for sedentary people was performed at the Cooper Aerobics Institute in Texas. A major part of their clinical operation is performing exercise tolerance tests to assess fitness levels in the employees sent by their corporate clients. The Institute then sets up an individual fitness program for the employee and reevaluates him or her every year. These subjects broke down into three groups:

- Fit (good exercise tolerance), who remained fit
- Unfit (low exercise tolerance), who remained unfit despite advice to exercise
- Unfit who became fit (performed the recommended exercise and improved the fitness levels on second and third return visits)

During the follow-up periods, the Institute obtained data on cardiac events and deaths, and found that the fit subjects had a much lower event rate than the unfit subjects (not surprising) and that *the unfit subjects who exercised and became fit had a much lower cardiac event and death rate than did the unfit subjects who did not follow the exercise recommendations and remained unfit.* An important finding was that the event-free survival curves began to diverge very early (by the next annual exam date) after the unfit patient was counseled. The yearly data plot suggested, in fact, that unfit patients who exercised effectively started to reduce their heart-event rate within months, and that the benefit, when compared to the continually unfit patients, increased every year!

Cardioprotective Impact of Regular Exercise on Sedentary Men

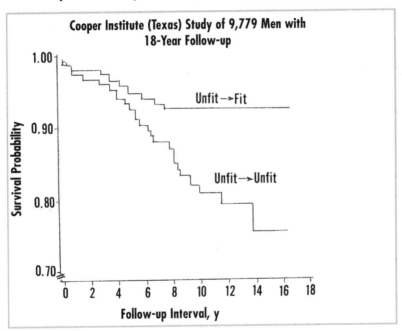

Exercise, then, is a proactive factor that you can use to reduce your heart attack risk, even in the presence of risk factors such as elevated cholesterol and smoking, and factors that you cannot change such as a family history of heart disease, or your own history of a heart attack or stroke.

HOW DOES EXERCISE WORK? (EXERCISE PHYSIOLOGY 101)

When you begin any exercise—walking on a treadmill, for example—your leg muscles start to do more work. To do this increased work they consume energy, which the body provides in the form of a high energy molecule called adenosine triphosphate, or ATP.

If our bodies were automobiles, ATP would be our gasoline!

The muscle cells make ATP by metabolizing, or "burning," small molecules of fats or sugars with oxygen, all of which are provided by the blood. As we walk faster and use more ATP, the muscle cells require more blood to produce more ATP. The heart responds to this increased need for blood by pumping harder to push more of it through the body to the muscles. The work being performed by our bodies is often measured by the number of calories of energy produced in the form of ATP to fuel the muscles. So when we say one mile of walking "burns" 100 calories, we mean that this amount of walking will require 100 calories from the metabolism of sugars and fats to produce the necessary amount of ATP to keep the muscles functioning.

As the heart beats faster and stronger to pump more blood to our muscles, the heart muscle itself is working harder and so it, in turn, needs an increased supply of blood. This blood is provided by the heart's own artery system, called the coronary arteries. If these arteries are partially blocked, as they are when you have atherosclerotic heart disease, then some of the heart muscle will require more oxygen-rich blood during exercise than the narrowed arteries can supply. We call this imbalance ischemia. Ischemia is often the first indication of heart disease, since it will often cause chest pain during exercise and will also show up as a change in your electrocardiogram on a stress test (doctors often refer to ischemia as having a "positive stress test"), or in the picture of your heart that doctors obtain in nuclear stress testing (often called a thallium stress test) or on stress echocardiogram that uses sonar technology to produce a moving picture of the walls of the beating heart.

When we exercise or "train" regularly, we increase the amount of exercise or work we can do and we actually lower the oxygen and blood requirement that the heart needs during exercise. This change is brought about by our trained body muscles being able to extract more oxygen from the blood that is pumped to them, and our heart increasing the amount of blood pumped with each beat.

Exercise physiology does not, however, tell us *why* we see fewer heart attacks and fewer instances of cardiac death in people with or without heart disease who exercise regularly. Until recently, the only factors we had identified that may have explained some of this reduction in heart disease with regular exercise are the increase of about 10 percent in the HDL (good) cholesterol and a small decrease in the clotting activity of our blood.

Now, our understanding of the function of the endothelial cell provides a logical explanation. The endothelial cells that line our blood vessels respond to the force of blood moving over its surface by producing nitric oxide. Nitric oxide causes the smooth muscle surrounding the artery to relax and the vessel to dilate. (See the Introduction for a discussion of how nitric oxide's effect on arteries and on atherosclerosis was discovered.) When we are exercising, the faster and stronger beating of the heart increases the forces on the endothelial cells. When exercise is done on a regular basis (as with exercise training or a regular exercise program), our endothelial cells "learn" to make more nitric oxide and to dilate more. When they dilate more, they also produce more small chemicals, called cytokines, which protect the artery from atherosclerosis and help to protect any atherosclerotic plaques that we have from fracturing, thus reducing heart attacks.

Characteristics of a Vulnerable Plaque

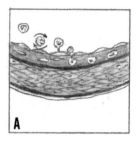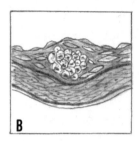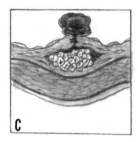

A   B   C

THE SYMPATHETIC/PARASYMPATHETIC EFFECT

Another mechanism of regular exercise that plays an important role in reducing cardiovascular death is the "turning down" of the sympathetic (fight-or-flight) nervous system activity and the increasing of the parasympathic, or vagal activity (rest and relaxation) on the heart. Studies have repeatedly shown that when the relative activity of these two systems is measured in patients with heart disease, the patients with the greatest parasympathetic activity have the best survival rates. Participating in regular exercise is one of the few things that you can do to change this balance for the better! We don't yet precisely know how this phenomenon works physiologically, but the consistent results of repeated studies convince us that it does. (For a fuller discussion of this effect, see New Rule No. 6 on the mind-body Connection to heart disease, beginning page 118.)

THE "BEST" EXERCISE? THE ONE YOU'LL STICK WITH!

Despite late-night TV infomercials for the latest wonderful exercise machine, there is no one "best" exercise. Only you can determine the "best" exercise: it's the one you will stick with on a regular basis throughout your life. There are, however, some basic principles of exercise training for cardiovascular health that have been gleaned from the studies of exercise and heart disease.

Do it aerobically

The exercise you choose should be mostly aerobic, meaning that the muscle cells generate most of their ATP by metabolizing fatty acids and sugars with an abundant supply of oxygen that results from a large increase in the amount of blood that the heart pumps each minute. Activities that promote this mechanism usually involve large movements of the legs or legs and arms in a repetitive fashion, against moderate to low resistance. Running, jogging, brisk walking, cycling, rowing, aerobics, dance, cross-country skiing, and using stepping machines and rowing machines are all examples of aerobic exercise.

Do it frequently

A contemporary analysis of the major published studies supported by the Office of the Surgeon General suggests performing aerobic exercise for 45 minutes to an hour three to five times a week.

Include resistance training

Although there are only a few studies suggesting the cardioprotective value of resistance training with weights or slow calisthenics, these studies are convincing about the satisfaction we feel in combining this training with aerobics. Resistance training provides the satisfaction from increasing muscle strength, which in turn reduces falls and injuries, and allows us to achieve a positive effect on our continued commitment to exercise. A good and balanced way to add resistance training to your program is to perform it twice a week, on nonaerobic exercise days, if you don't exercise aerobically every day.

Resistance training protocols were originally developed to increase strength and muscle size to the maximum extent attainable. The usual format was a "set" of exercises that isolate individual muscle groups, performed with enough weight to permit only six to eight repetitions (referred to as "reps") before you could not do it again (called "working to failure"). This set was repeated three times in a workout (three sets). When you were able to do more than eight reps easily, you increased the weight to bring your working-to-failure number of repetitions down to six.

Strength training experiments have changed this format. Performing eight to ten repetitions to fatigue (near failure, not failure) once (one set), working out 10 to 12 major muscle groups (arms, legs, chest, abdomen, and back), will achieve 80 percent of the strength achieved in the traditional protocol outlined above. This new format will also reduce the time, discomfort, and injuries involved, and enhance your chances of staying with it. Two good ways to do this new protocol are to use a set of adjustable dumbbells, a bench, and a mat, as well as good instruction from a trainer or instructor; or to use a multistation strength training machine setup. Here, too, instruction and supervision as you get started will reduce injury and optimize results and satisfaction.

Do it intensely

Intensity is important during any exercise routine, since the greatest increase in training effect occurs with an exercise that is performed at greater than 60 percent of our maximum exercise capacity. This level of intensity is also necessary to perform the quantity of work in terms of calories burned that will significantly reduce your risk of a heart attack.

MEASURING INTENSITY

Exercise heart rates should be in the 60 to 80 percent of maximum heart rate range. There are two methods of ascertaining that you are performing aerobic exercise activities at the appropriate level of intensity. One method forces you to rely on equipment and complicated math formulas to determine your maximum heart rate. This method is outlined in the box on the next page. The method that most people find most useful, and the one I recommend, is called the Rate of Perceived Exertion.

Rate of Perceived Exertion (RPE)

This method, developed by Dr. Gunnar Borg in Sweden, is based on the notion that your mind "knows" how much exercise your body is doing. Dr. Borg's original scale went from 6 (no effort, at rest) to 22 (maximal effort, exhaustion). When subjects used this scale, their answers were very close to more "scientific" measures of how much work they were doing and how hard their hearts were working.

An even more useful version of the RPE scale is from one to ten, making it easy to teach and remember (see Appendix II). Simply put, when you feel that you are exercising at a seven or eight on this scale, you are very close to the 70 to 80 percent of your maximum exercise intensity, and, in most cases, closer than you would be if you used the other methods, which are based on your "target" pulse rate while you exercise.

Another benefit of using the RPE technique is that you can "take it with you" as you try different activities or where it is difficult to measure your pulse, such as when you are swimming. I teach RPE to all my patients.

Duration

There is no clear evidence that any specific length of time during which we exercise achieves the greatest training effect or the

---

MEASURING YOUR MAXIMUM AND TARGET HEART RATES

Your target pulse rate—the number of beats per minute your heart should be beating during a workout—is determined as a percentage (usually 60 to 80 percent) of your maximum heart rate. This maximum value can be determined accurately only during a supervised exercise EKG examination that measures your pulse rate at your highest exercise level. For example, if your peak heart rate near exhaustion during your treadmill test is 160, your exercise heart rate range should be 112 to 128.

This formula works well *only* when you have an actual measurement of your maximum heart rate. If you use an estimate of your maximum heart rate, from the commonly used equation *Maximum Heart Rate = 220 − your age,* you will be off your real peak heart rate by an amount sufficient to make the calculated training heart rate too low (below 60 percent peak) or too high (above 80 to 85 percent peak) a large percentage of the time. My advice is to use the RPE method instead.

Patients with heart disease who have taken an exercise EKG examination to near exhaustion will learn their real maximum heart rate. For these individuals I can recommend a target heart rate of 60 to 80 percent of this measured near-maximum rate with confidence. A wrist-watch device (one good brand is Polar) that monitors heart rate is an excellent method of monitoring exercise intensity.

highest level of cardiac protection. In fact, the fastest increases among athletes in aerobic training programs occur with very short intervals of exercise separated by short intervals of rest. Three-minute bursts of exercise followed by one-minute rest intervals increase exercise capacity faster than any other protocol, but it is not a particularly satisfying, pleasant, or realistic way to exercise. For most of us, exercising for 40 minutes three to five times a week, or one-half hour of aerobics every day, with an additional activity (resistance training, for instance) twice a week for an additional half hour, will achieve a rapid and significant training effect and will place us in the cardioprotective range. Another equally reasonable approach is to do three 10-minute exercise sessions a day with a fixed 30-minute session twice a week. The 10 minutes during the day can be a brisk walk to work, or the last part of your trip to work, a brisk walk at lunch time, and a moderately vigorous bike ride at the end of the day. Whatever works best for you is right!

Avoiding Injury

Injury is the biggest risk to losing the protective value of a regular exercise program. Injuries most often occur because of too rapid an increase in intensity or duration that results in muscle soreness or joint or back pain. We think we should stop exercising until we feel better and then return to the program at a lower level of intensity, but I find commonly that a patient's response to injury is to wait until the pain is gone and then not return to exercise. Minor injuries are a major reason that exercise programs fail.

The following are some do's and don'ts gleaned from my patients and from experience with my own exercise programs and injuries:

1. Slowly increase duration or intensity of aerobic exercise, and start resistance training slowly. If possible, seek the advice of a trainer or physical education instructor.

2. Select an activity with a low-risk profile and setting. Jogging and bicycle riding are great aerobic activities, but must be done safely. When running, choose a well-lighted, moderately soft, safe, and even surface without problems in the ground that could make you fall. Don't do outdoor exercises, such as bike riding, at dusk or at night. Wearing a reflective vest will protect you from cars, but not from tripping or falling on a hidden ridge or hole in the ground. Outdoor exercise is always best done with a partner. Avoid dangerous, hilly, poorly lit settings.

3. Wear the right gear! This is important not only to "look the part" but because the right shoes will provide support, traction, and shock absorption. The properly fitted bicycle will allow a comfortable riding posture and seat height, and the correct eye protection, head gear or helmet, and wrist and knee protection when appropriate can be the difference between a nasty fall and a tragedy.

4. Don't pick exercise as a way to fulfill a fantasy! I see many men with back and hamstring problems who choose to get their exercise by starting karate or kickboxing lessons and women who go back to the dance training of their younger years. You can engage in these activities if you work with a skilled instructor and at an age-appropriate level. But don't expect to step up quickly to your remembered levels or you will risk injury as well as, probably, disappointment.

5. Warm up and cool down? The data are actually pretty

soft. There is clear evidence that athletes who exercise before a competition will perform better. One study showed that competitive swimmers who warmed up by doing practice laps had faster times than they did when they competed without a warm-up. But there is no data from well-designed studies that document a reduction in injuries or postexercise soreness. However, the experience of coaches, trainers, and athletes strongly suggests that warming up and cooling down are good ideas. A good "investment" in your program is to warm up by initiating the exercise activity slowly and building up to the training intensity over three to five minutes, then cooling down for the same period at the end and stretching some injury-prone muscle groups after exercise. The rationale for stretching "warm" muscles and tendons is that the stretch will be more effective than when stretching "cold" before exercise. Bottom line is: stretching is probably helpful, but if you hate it, you can skip it. (I know that some very respected trainers and exercise class leaders will strongly disagree with this advice!)

6. Get advice and help early. If you wait for pain to get worse, it usually will. Sometimes the best advice can come from an athletic trainer who is very knowledgeable about your activity. An excellent running coach may often be more helpful than your doctor regarding techniques of running and training to reduce injuries or pain. A knowledgeable physical therapist can be of exceptional value. Seek the recommendation of a good physical therapist from someone who regularly engages in your sport. For serious pain, that is, pain that persists and is made worse by the exercise, see the appropriate physician,

frequently a sports medicine specialist or an orthopedic surgeon.

THE REAL RISK VS. BENEFIT OF EXERCISE

The first part of this chapter presented the data supporting the remarkable protection against heart attacks afforded by a regular, moderately vigorous aerobic exercise program involving three to five sessions a week and paired with a strength-training program performed twice a week. But those of you who have coronary disease may be afraid of starting a program, and I want to address the risk of having a heart attack or other serious cardiac event by doing vigorous exercise.

The first reported case of sudden death following an extraordinary athletic feat is that of Phaedippas, the father of the contemporary marathon who, as told by Thucydides, died suddenly after running the 26 miles from the plains of Marathon to the city of Athens to report victory against Persian invaders. In more recent times, marathons, other physical events, and all forms of aerobic exercise have been associated with rare but well publicized episodes of heart attacks and sudden death. In almost all cases, the deaths occurred in people who had coronary heart disease and, in many instances, were exercising at a level of intensity, or in a temperature or at an altitude beyond that to which they were accustomed. However, it is clear that vigorous exercise represents a small risk to heart patients. Several studies in the past decade have made it possible to put this risk in perspective vis à vis the cardioprotective gains, and have suggested ways to minimize any risk.

One study by Dr. Paul Thompson and colleagues on joggers in Rhode Island reported that the absolute risk of sudden death or heart attack is very small: one death for every 396,000 hours of exercise. This statistic was placed in perspective by the Myocardial Infarction Onset Study, reported in 1995. Specially trained nurses interviewed patients who entered emergency units of participating hospitals with a heart attack within 24 hours of their admission. They asked the patients to account for each hour of the 24 hours prior to their coronary event and recorded the patients' recall of any physical and emotional events they experienced. Then the patient was asked to recall the day 48 hours prior to the heart attack (for example, if the heart attack occurred on Friday, they were also asked to detail their activities for the same time period on Wednesday). Events that were more common on the heart attack than the non–heart attack day were considered to have played a role in triggering the heart attack. The nurses asked the patients if they exercised regularly and, if so, how often they did so in a week?

The events that occurred more often on the day of the heart attack, and indeed in the 2 hours before a heart attack, were:

- a period of vigorous exercise that was more than the person was accustomed to,
- sexual intercourse, or
- intense emotional episodes (either angry or happy).

These events were considered to have played a role in triggering the heart attack. The important protective role of regular exercise was evident in the finding that the risk of a session of vigorous exercise precipitating a heart attack was lost (that is, near zero!) in the patient who regularly exercised more than three times a week. Not only was regular vigorous exercise protective in its own right, but it seemed to protect these patients from the risk of the vigorous exercise session itself causing a heart attack.

The lesson here? Once you get into a regular exercise program, then the risk of each exercise session causing a heart attack is less and less. In other words, if you are aerobically fit, the risk of having a heart attack during an exercise session is much lower than even the very low risk of a heart attack when you are unfit and decide to have an exercise session.

The bottom line? Start slowly, so you're not doing a lot of vigorous exercise you aren't accustomed to doing, and build up over a period of weeks or months, so that you are getting two, three, four, five sessions a week of vigorous exercise. This way, you are never so far ahead in your fitness that you are putting an unaccustomed strain on the heart. As you build up the exercise session time and intensity to three-plus times a week, not only do your heart and your muscles become more efficient, but you stabilize your plaque as well. The process is wonderful! The more blood flowing over your endothelial cells as you exercise regularly, the more nitric oxide and other beneficial chemicals the cells produce, the more relaxed the blood vessels remain, and finally, the less likely the blood vessels are to develop plaques or to have those plaques fracture and cause a heart attack.

Being fit also protects you from an increase in heart attack risk when you do unaccustomed exercise, such as running up a hill to the station to catch a train, or across the airline terminal with your baggage to catch a plane, or shoveling snow. One very important protective effect of regular exercise noted in the Myocardial Infarction Onset Study was that the risk of a heart attack being triggered by sexual intercourse was, while low in everyone, even lower in patients who exercise regularly.

ONE MORE IMPORTANT STEP TO REDUCE THE RISK IN STARTING AN EXERCISE PROGRAM

There is, however, more to reducing your risk of exercise triggering a heart attack than just careful and gradual increases in the training program. We must avoid starting a vigorous exercise session when there is significant disease in our coronary arteries that we know about or, more often, that we are unaware of. A prudent approach to reduce this risk involves an examination by your doctor and very possibly a stress test (see New Rule No. 8, beginning page 165, on determining the best tests for you) if you fit into any of the following categories:

- You have diabetes or a strong first-order-relative history of early heart disease
- You have a history of smoking, high LDL cholesterol, or high blood pressure
- You exhibit symptoms that may be angina pectoris (chest pain or pressure on exertion or stress, or some-times—especially in women—extreme fatigue, or sweat-ing, or burning midline chest pain)
- Your EKG shows an abnormality

For a more complete discussion of cardiac risk factors, see New Rule No. 2, beginning on page 26.

If you have not exercised regularly and have these risk factors, symptoms, or associated medical conditions, you and your doc-tor must investigate further to determine if you have coronary artery disease, before you begin a new exercise regime. Rule out any cardiac problems before hitting the gym or jogging trail.

THE NEW RULES EXERCISE PROGRAM

1. *Getting Started:* Start walking 20 minutes a day at a comfortable but brisk pace. Use the RPE method to set your intensity at 5 or 6 out of 10. This can be done as two 10-minute walks on a relatively flat surface (no

steep hills!). Wear comfortable shoes or sneakers. This is the preliminary activity and can be started today.

2. Decide if you need to see your doctor, that is, if you have heart disease or you have the symptoms described in New Rule No. 1, beginning on page 17, or are at moderate risk or greater as calculated in New Rule No. 2, beginning on page 26. At this point, you might possibly need to have a stress test to detect signs of previously unknown heart disease.

3. Pick your aerobic exercise and the location at which you'll perform it. Select and solicit your partner(s) if appropriate—one of the best favors you can do for yourself and your friends—and invest in a good pair of cross-trainers or running shoes. Select comfortable clothing that is appropriate for the exercise. Expense here is for your head only (which, as we noted, can be important), as the heart doesn't know if you are working out in designer togs or your old sweats. Remember: Convenience and safety are critical issues in exercising aerobically.

4. Start slowly and work up in a gradual manner. A good rule of thumb that professional trainers use is to increase intensity and duration by less than 10 percent every two to three weeks at the most. Remember: success here is not rapidly achieving elevated intensity or duration but finding a pleasant and rewarding program that you stick to.

5. Use the RPE method to regulate intensity, with a level of six or seven as a good working goal. As you train you will increase your intensity automatically by staying at this RPE score. This is one of beautiful things about this method!

6. Exercise for 30 to 45 minutes three to seven days a

week. If you select a 45-minute workout in a gym or an aerobics class, then three times a week is ideal. If you are walking briskly for 30 minutes, try to include most if not all days of the week.

7. Sports physiologists and coaches recommend spending two to three minutes "warming up" to your exercise speed and stride, and the same time slowing down as you approach the end of your session. Warming up and cooling down will likely make you feel better at the end of each exercise session.

8. If you feel mild muscle soreness or back pain, cut back on RPE for two weeks to see if the symptoms improve, and then go back to level six or seven. If you are in a supervised facility, such as a gym or health club, ask the professional trainers for some things you can do to get rid of the symptoms. Try not to stop completely unless the pain is moderately intense or persists for more than a few days. In this case, seek immediate help. (Sports-knowledgeable physicians, orthopedic surgeons or physiatrists, or a physical therapist are the best choices here.)

Stick with this beginning program for the first two weeks. During this time, check with your doctor about any concerns you may have and have appropriate testing performed if you meet the criteria outlined in New Rules No. 1 (imminent heart attack) and 2 (long-term risk factors).

If there are any issues that your doctor thinks should be addressed regarding your medical condition, then attend to them now. Assuming there are no heart or other issues that your physician thinks should impact an exercise program, you should design and start your exercise program as follows:

Select your main exercise activity. This should be aerobic, and allow for varying intensity and duration. In order of importance, the choice should be made on the following factors: (1) Pick the exercise you prefer, not what you think is the best exercise—you most likely will not do it otherwise. (2) Choose an activity that is convenient, flexible with regard to time or partners, and not too expensive. Again you will most likely stop exercise if these criteria are not met. (3) Consider safety. Don't run alone in an isolated area or choose an activity that lends itself to injury. (4) Address prior injuries or conditions, such as arthritis, that cause pain during or after exercise. Check with your physician and an exercise specialist, such as a staff member at your Y or gym or a professional exercise trainer, to select an activity that will not result in pain, and include activities that will improve your muscle or joint problems.

Start with 15 to 20 minutes and work up by adding 5 minutes every two to four weeks to reach 30 to 45 minutes.

Use the RPE method to control intensity unless you have had a maximum stress test and have been given a "target heart rate," in which case you should monitor your target heart rate with a heart rate watch. (Polar is a popular brand that my patients have found very satisfactory.)

Add 5 minutes of upper body calisthenics per exercise session if you have chosen an activity that uses legs only, such as walking or jogging.

Do resistance training twice a week with hand weights (dumbbells) or muscle-specific machines at a gym or spa. If you use the machines, have your program set up according to the following criteria by a trained staff member at the facility. If you are using hand weights at home, follow these general rules: Do each activity at the weight or resistance that will cause you to stop from fatigue at 10 repetitions. As you train, the exercise will get easier, so increase the weight by small amounts (1 to 2 pounds for arm and hand activities) to keep yourself "tired at 10." Remember that resistance training twice a week, each time with one set of 10 reps that exercise the arms, legs, shoulders, hips, abdomen, and back (about 8 to 10 activities) is what you need. If the activity hurts, stop and get expert advice. You may be holding your body and doing the exercise (especially with the dumbbells) incorrectly. You may need to select a different activity or start at a lower weight or resistance.

Add a team sport or hiking to your activities whenever you can. They will allow you to enjoy your fitness and agility, and keep up your motivation. Nothing succeeds like success.

Involve family and friends in this program with some or all of your activities. Their participation will help you stay on track and you will be doing them an enormous favor by increasing their fitness level and allowing them to stave off heart disease. Remind them that their participation in your exercise routine is your gift to them that keeps on giving!

EAT WELL: MINIMAL DIET GUIDELINES FOR MAXIMUM HEART-HEALTH BENEFITS

In medical school, what I (and most doctors of my generation) learned about nutrition could fill just a paragraph of one chapter in this book. A very short paragraph. What I learned had to do with infant nutrition during my pediatrics rotation, something about the timing of switching a baby from formula to solid foods, and which solid foods to introduce. End of nutrition instruction in medical school!

Yet, as the role of cholesterol in the development of athero-sclerosis was studied and better understood, doctors viewed the role of nutrition in maintaining heart health as increasingly important. Many different diets were proposed, tested, and pub-lished. In this chapter I outline the basic information you need to know about what to eat to outlive heart disease.

A heart-healthy eating plan does not have to be complicated. I recommend a modified version of the DASH (Dietary Approaches to Stop Hypertension) diet, originally developed to control high blood pressure, but now thought to be the basis of the best, tastiest, and most balanced eating plan for almost everyone. The rules are pretty simple and your best chance of "winning" the battle with heart disease is to play by the New Rules!

A BIT OF DIET HISTORY

During my cardiology training, the role of cholesterol in the development of atherosclerosis was becoming an increasingly important subject to understand, but relatively little was known about the role nutrition plays in the prevention and treatment of heart disease. One event in my earlier medical training stands out in my mind. The medical library at Kings County Hospital in Brooklyn was named the Doc Library in honor of the former chief of the medical service, Dr. William Doc. During my chief residency in medicine, I was assigned to escort Dr. Doc, who had been invited to return as a visiting professor. Lunch conference in the Doc Library was an important part of the day and I rounded up the interns and residents to hear his presentation and to present their most interesting and difficult cases for his comments and suggestions. Dr. Doc, an energetic man in his eighties, shared with me that he had suffered a heart attack six months previously, and was treating himself based on some of the early animal studies on diet and exercise and atherosclerosis that he had done as a young doctor. He said he now walked 20 to 30 blocks in New York City every day, climbed the six flights to his apartment instead of using the elevator, and ate a near-vegetarian diet. While the residents and I had our usual medical conference lunch of Coca-Cola and pizza, he opened his Tupperware container and lunched on pieces of fresh fruits, nuts, and lightly cooked vegetables. In retrospect, it was impressive that he was so far ahead of the prevailing practices about a healthy diet.

Today we know much more about the role of diet in preventing and treating heart disease and why it is an essential part of a plan to outlive it. The scientific studies that have made the case for a heart-healthy diet include those that examine the eating habits of citizens of countries with higher rates of heart attacks compared with the eating habits of people from countries with lower rates of heart attacks. There are also studies that include clinical trials with patients assigned at random to the study diet or their usual diets. In some cases, these trials have shown a very significant reduction in second heart attacks and heart complications in patients assigned to the specific study diet.

THE SEVEN COUNTRIES STUDY AND FOLLOW-UP

One of the most important studies that caused us to rethink the role of nutrition in the development of heart disease was the Seven Countries Study and its recent 25-year follow-up report. This study, which began in 1954, looked at groups of men in Italy, Greece, Yugoslavia, Finland, the Netherlands, Japan, and the United States, and recorded their incidence of heart disease as well as their known risk factors such as smoking, high blood pressure, and elevated blood cholesterol. It also looked at diet. Seven Countries showed us that men living near the Mediterranean Sea (Italy, Greece) and in the Pacific Rim (Japan) had many fewer heart attacks than those living in northern Europe and the United States. The major differences between the two groups were their diets and their blood cholesterol levels, and researchers began to show a link between the two. Countries with high heart attack rates (northern Europe and the United States) had diets high in saturated fats—fats found in meat, whole-milk foods (such as cream, most cheeses, and—my favorite—ice cream) and some vegetable oils (such as palm and coconut). Men from these countries also had increased blood cholesterol levels.

> As noted in earlier chapters, women were not included in many of the early studies of the development of heart disease because it was thought to be rare in women at that time.

An important question remained: was heart attack risk strictly about the effect of the foods we eat on our cholesterol levels? If it were, we could, in theory, eat whatever we choose and use cholesterol-lowering drugs (such as the statins) to keep our cholesterol down and still avoid heart disease. My personal food fantasy in this regard is a rich vanilla ice cream (Häagen-Dazs) bar covered with a crunchy almond and chocolate-flavored statin!

The Seven Countries 25-year follow-up study answered this question: No. Diet is not strictly about its effect on blood cholesterol. How do we know this? The data clearly showed that a man with a total cholesterol level of 250mg/dl living in a Mediterranean country on a diet rich in seafood, fresh fruits, vegetables, and olive oil had *not quite half* the chance of dying of heart disease than his northern European counterparts with the same cholesterol level whose diet was high in saturated fats from meat, dairy products, and animal and vegetable shortening. This finding was true even after such risk factors as smoking and high blood pressure were accounted for. *Diet has a direct and important role in heart disease that goes beyond cholesterol,* and although we may, in the future, discover the many important mechanisms behind a high-risk diet and develop drugs to reverse them, we cannot now or in the near future eat a typical northern European or U.S. diet and avoid heart disease just by lowering our cholesterol.

THE HEART-HEALTHY MEDITERRANEAN DIET

Looking at countries with low risks of heart attack, the Seven Countries investigators noted important similarities in their diets when compared with the high-risk countries. The diets in Italy and Greece, where the rate of heart disease was low, had these elements in common:

- Less fat and much less saturated fat than northern European and U.S. diets
- More fruits, vegetables, nuts, seeds, and whole grains food servings every week
- Two or more fish meals a week
- More olive oil used for food preparation
- Fewer servings of whole milk dairy products
- One or two glasses of wine a day
- Total caloric intake per day better matched to the calories used in daily activity, resulting in less obesity

This combination of foods and lifestyle was termed a "Mediterranean diet," since the countries were on or near the Mediterranean Sea. This low-risk diet was the basis of a second group of studies, the most important of which was the Lyon Diet Heart Study, which addressed this question: will a low heart-risk diet help patients with heart disease to have fewer second heart attacks and live longer?

In the Lyon Diet Heart Study, investigators researched the effect of a Mediterranean-type diet with the addition of a special margarine developed from canola oil that was rich in a specific unsaturated fat called alpha linolenic acid, often referred to as ALA. ALA is the fat found in some seeds and vegetable oils and is similar to the heart-healthy fats found in fish and fish oil. In all, 302 heart patients were placed on the Lyon diet (and an equal number of patients in a control group continued to eat their usual diet). The patients were studied over a five-year period. The outcome, published in 1999, was astounding! The researchers found a 76 percent reduction in cardiac deaths in the diet intervention group when compared with the control group. Patients on this special Mediterranean diet had less than one-quarter the chance of having a second heart attack than the patients who ate their regular diet, despite the fact that both groups were on medication therapy, such as statins, to lower cholesterol!

Diet clearly is a powerful tool for lowering one's risk of developing coronary artery disease and for living longer with fewer heart problems if you already have heart disease.

THE NEW RULES–RECOMMENDED DIET? THE DASH DIET

Is there one best diet?

Similar to my recommendation in the previous chapter regarding your exercise program, the best diet is one that you will stick with, which means that, in addition to being heart healthy, it must be easy to shop for and prepare, tasty to your palate, adaptable at most restaurants, and easily customized to your family's food preferences. A heart-healthy diet must also be the basis of an effective and enduring weight reduction and maintenance program, since heart attack risk increases significantly when you are overweight or obese. (See the previous chapter about assessing your risk factors for developing heart disease.)

The diet that I and many of my colleagues follow and recommend to our patients is based on the Mediterranean diet, specifically a version of this diet modified for the foods, tastes, and budgets of people in the United States. It was developed and tested as a diet to help prevent and control high blood pressure, but it also has benefits that keep your heart healthy. Its name: the DASH diet.

The DASH diet grew out of a diet intervention study developed to lower blood pressure in those patients who were suffering from hypertension. It is very similar to a Mediterranean diet regarding the amount of protein, carbohydrates (sugars), and fats, and the actual foods from which you derive these nutrients, including the amount of saturated and unsaturated fats allowed. DASH differs from the Mediterranean diet in that it calls for two to three more servings a day of fruits and vegetables. These extra servings increase the diet's potassium, calcium, and magnesium, which are minerals called electrolytes.

Another electrolyte that is reduced in the DASH diet is sodium, which finds its way into our diet as salt. We get salt not only from the table salt we may use in preparing food or as a taste enhancer before eating, but as a key ingredient in many common prepared foods. (Big Macs and most canned soups are loaded with sodium.) The DASH diet's extra fruit and vegetable servings also increase the amount of fiber that we eat every day; fiber is helpful in lowering our cholesterol in our bloodstream, helping us to feel full on less food, and keeping our bowels in good working order.

One legitimate question to ask is this: if I don't have high blood pressure, should I still follow the DASH diet? The answer is yes, because it is a perfect Mediterranean diet and all of us stand a good chance of developing high blood pressure as we age. A recent analysis of blood pressure data from the Framingham study (see New Rule No. 2 on risk factors) found that 80 percent of the men and women in that group who had normal blood pressure at age 60 developed high blood pressure eventually. This finding moved the DASH diet from a specialty diet to treat high blood pressure to a diet of importance to everyone. Designed specifically for this purpose, the DASH diet may not only help to limit the rise in blood pressure, but will decrease your chances of developing heart disease.

> For a small number of people with kidney disease or who are on drugs that tend to raise blood potassium levels, the extra potassium in the DASH diet may be a concern. In this case, some of the fruit servings should be changed to servings of vegetables with a low amount of potassium, such as asparagus, carrots, cauliflower, corn, eggplant, green beans, green peas, and squash. Ask your doctor if this is a concern for you. If it is, you should receive special dietary instructions.

SEEING IS BELIEVING: THE NEW RULES VERSION OF THE DASH DIET

The following is a serving list and a sample menu for the New Rules version of the DASH diet. I find that this kind of list and sample menu is the only way to visualize what you would be eating when following the diet.

> Portion control, in the DASH diet and in any heart-healthy diet, is key. Correct portions are the following:
>
> - Meat, poultry, and fish servings are 3 ounces (about the size of a deck of playing cards)
> - Grains servings are 1 slice of bread (preferably whole grain), ½ cup of rice or pasta
> - Milk (preferably skim milk) is an 8-ounce glass or 1 cup of yogurt

New Rules–Modified DASH DIET
Daily Serving List

Food Group	Servings per Day at about 2,000 cal/day
Grains/grain products	8 per day
Vegetables	5
Fruits	3
Low fat/fat-free dairy*	4–5
Meat, poultry, fish[†]	1–2 per day
Nuts, seeds, dried beans[‡]	1
Fats/oils[§]	2–3
Sweets	0
Soy (milk, tofu, cheese)	1–2

*If you are lactase-deficient (have too little of the enzyme that breaks down the sugar in milk and find that milk produces cramps and diarrhea), or if you don't like dairy products, you can substitute both of the dairy servings with soy milk, tofu, or soy cheeses, or take two calcium supplement tablets. The New Rules version of the DASH diet calls for everyone to eat one to two soy servings a day, because soy proteins lower cholesterol; soy also contains isoflavones, which are rich in the antioxidants known to have a role in reducing a necessary step in the formation of plaques in our blood vessels.

[†]In order to get the benefit of the omega-3 oils you will need to eat two servings of fish a week. The problem here is the high level of mercury and other toxins, such as PCPs, found in many fish, including tile fish, shark, swordfish, and farm-bred salmon. (Most of the salmon in the United States is, unfortunately, bred in ocean water fish farms.) The USDA recommends that pregnant women avoid many types of fish and that most people limit fish meals to twice a week. An alternative that I recommend is to eat one fish meal a week and take one fish oil capsule per

New Rules–Modified DASH Diet Sample Menu

BREAKFAST

A fresh fruit (navel orange)—6 oz.

1% low-fat or skim milk or soy milk—8 oz.

Oat or bran cereal with 1 tsp. sugar—1 cup

---

day (usually in the form of one-gram capsules that are widely available). The fish oil capsules should state on their label that the fish oil has been tested to be free of mercury. ALA, which provides many of the benefits of omega-3 oils, is also an alternative to fish and fish oils. Another alternative is a synthetically produced (from ocean plants) form of the fish oil DHA.

†Eating one-quarter cup of raw or dry roasted nuts, preferably almonds and walnuts, although peanuts are okay, three or more times a week is an excellent idea. The oils (fats) in nuts are rich in ALA and have been shown to lower LDL cholesterol and to have a variety of other heart-healthy benefits. Remember, though, that nuts are very high in calories. One-quarter cup of nuts is about 170 calories, so portion control is a must.

§Three products to emphasize in the fats and oils category are olive oil or canola oil and a margarine that contains stanols and sterols. Stanols are the vegetable version of the cholesterol our bodies manufacture, and when we eat them, we lower our LDL cholesterol. Also, sprinkle a tablespoon of flaxseed over a salad or a vegetable serving. The flaxseed, and to a lesser extent the canola, provide the important ALA—the vegetable omega-3 fatty acids.

Note: An excellent presentation of the DASH diet (without my New Rules modifications) is available free from the National Heart, Lung, and Blood Institute information center (www.nhbli.nih.gov).

Whole grain bread with 1 tsp. jelly—1 slice
Soft margarine with stanols—1 tsp.

LUNCH

Turkey breast or chicken salad—3 oz. or ¾ cup
Whole grain roll—2-inch in diameter
Raw vegetable medley: carrot and celery sticks, lettuce, green or
  red pepper slices—about ½ to ¾ cup
Part-skim mozzarella cheese or tofu or soy cheese—either one
  stick *or* 1½ slices
Fresh fruit or baked apple (baked with sugar substitute)—1

DINNER

Herbed baked cod or other fish—3 oz.
Brown rice with scallions—1 cup
Steamed broccoli—½ cup
Stewed tomatoes—½ cup
Spinach salad with raw spinach, and fresh sliced tomatoes and
  l-inch cubes of tofu—1 cup sprinkled with:
    1 Tbsp. flaxseed
    Salad dressing with 1 tsp. olive or canola oil and balsamic
    vinegar
Whole grain baguette—2-inch-thick slice
Soft margarine with stanols—1 tsp.
Fruit dessert (melon with fresh strawberries or raspberries)—
  about ½ cup

SNACKS

Dried fruits—1 oz.
Nuts (raw or dry roasted almonds)—¼ cup
Tea—1 or more cups without sugar (use sugar substitute)

Note: If you are eating at a restaurant, it is nearly impossible to get a three-ounce serving of meat, poultry, or fish. A good way to start is to ask for half a serving (or share your serving with someone dining with you). Also, to avoid highly fattening dressings or sauces, ask that these be omitted or served on the side.

THE NEW RULES QUICK COURSE IN NUTRITIONAL SCIENCE—YES, YOU DO NEED TO READ THIS SECTION!

In order to understand why the DASH diet is so good for us, we need to look at the way that our bodies use nutrients, and understand why the fad diets you may have heard of to control weight don't deliver a heart-healthy way to do it. I'll also outline a simple method to determine whether you are overweight, and just how overweight you may be, by measuring your BMI.

Perhaps no area of medicine is the subject of more media attention than is our diet. Foods that are newly found to be good or bad for you, or special combinations of foods that will help you lose weight, improve energy, increase mental sharpness, or enhance sexual performance and prevent disease are always news. The result is that we are constantly bombarded with information that may be misleading and in many instances is just wrong. The only defense I know of against this barrage is the basic knowledge regarding nutrition that follows.

Macronutrients

There are only three major types of foods, termed macronutrients, that we eat to metabolize for energy or for use as building blocks that we need to build up and repair our bodies. These are as follows:

Proteins. Proteins are composed of small molecules called amino acids that can be metabolized to produce energy and are used by the body to synthesize most of its critical structural and chemical components. *Calories:* Proteins produce four kilocalories (the word we mean when we say "calories") per gram. Protein should not exceed 20 percent of the overall calories in your diet.

Carbohydrates. Often called sugars (although the sugar that we put in our tea or coffee is actually a specific type of carbohydrate called sucrose), carbohydrates exist as simple sugars or complex carbohydrates. Simple sugars are found in fruit juices, some vegetables, honey and maple syrup, and of course table sugar, and as the starch in potatoes, wheat, and rice. They are rapidly absorbed across the walls of our intestines and increase the glucose concentration in our blood. Complex carbohydrates, on the other hand, require further metabolic breakdown in our digestive system before we can absorb them; complex carbohydrates cause our blood sugar to rise more slowly than do simple carbohydrates. *Calories:* Carbohydrates produce four calories per gram of energy, and in most instances complex are better for us than simple.

Fats. The types of food we call fats are actually made up of chains of fatty acids. Depending on the chemical structure of the fatty acid, fats are termed saturated fatty acids (SFA), monounsaturated fatty acids (MUFA), or polyunsaturated fatty acids (PUFA). SFAs raise cholesterol the most, whereas MUFAs and PUFAs help to lower cholesterol. A fatty acid that is manufactured, not by nature, but by modern food production methods, is a transfat. We create transfats when we transform them with hydrogen to make them solid at room temperature, as we did with corn oil after World War II to produce the first margarines. Transfats raise LDL cholesterol to the same or an even greater extent than do saturated fats and should be avoided in our diets.

Calories: Fats are the richest source of energy, producing nine calories per gram.

Micronutrients

This term is used to refer to smaller molecules that are not usually sources of energy but play critical roles in our body's function. Micronutrients include vitamins, minerals, and other chemicals. One such class of chemicals is flavanoids, which are found in fruits, soy, vegetables, and nuts and act as antioxidants in our bodies. As previously noted, antioxidants in the food we eat may help prevent or stop atherosclerosis, since they may serve to inhibit an early stage of the disease that involves the oxidation of LDL cholesterol.

BALANCING THE MACRONUTRIENTS, FOODS TYPES, AND MICRONUTRIENTS: WHAT YOU NEED TO KNOW

Fat

Total fat consumption, measured as a percentage of the total number of calories we eat each day, should be at or below 30 percent. Less than 10 percent of total calories (about one-third of our fats) should be saturated fats and the remainder should be mono- and polyunsaturated fats. A higher percentage of saturated fats in our diets will increase cholesterol levels. A heart-healthy diet should include no transfats.

Proteins

Only 15 to 20 percent of our daily calories should come from proteins in our diet. More protein consumption may stress our kidneys.

Carbohydrates

The remainder of our calories (50 to 60 percent) should come from carbohydrates, mostly complex carbohydrates from foods like vegetables, whole grains, and fresh fruits, as opposed to the simple sugars in soda, candy, or syrups. Eating complex carbohydrates will minimize repeated rapid surges in blood sugar and the demand for high levels of insulin secretion by our pancreas. This relationship of the fats and carbohydrates in our diet (high fat content, lower carbohydrate and low-fat complex carbohydrates) is an important one when we look at some of the popular diets. The low-fat Ornish diet has only 10 percent of calories from fat and is a very high-carbohydrate diet—70 percent of calories are derived from carbohydrates. The Atkins diet, with 40 percent of calories from fat, has only 40 percent of its calories from carbohydrates. On a long-term basis, these extreme diets don't make good "heart sense."

Micronutrients

Micronutrients such as vitamins and minerals, and antioxidants such as flavanoids, are provided by seven to nine servings of fruits and vegetables a day. Supplements are not required and since supplements are not regulated by the FDA, they may even be risky. My one exception is a single multivitamin and mineral pill from a known and creditable company. A multivitamin may be of some value and represents no risk so long as you choose, if you are over age 45, one *without iron*, usually referred to as a "senior" or "silver" vitamin and mineral supplement.

Fiber

The American Heart Association diets recommend 25 to 30 grams of fiber from food each day, about twice the amount in the average American diet. Fiber from oats, beans, or phylum (a bulk laxative powder) is characterized as soluble fiber (meaning it dissolves in water and will lower LDL cholesterol) and insoluble fiber. The food servings that will achieve this recommended amount of fiber include eight servings of whole grain products, six servings of fruits or vegetables, and one serving of dried beans or legumes each day. Other good sources of soluble fiber include legumes and dried peas. Fruits, vegetables, and barley are a source of both types of fiber. It is suggested that you increase fiber in your diet in a gradual manner to avoid flatulence and bloating. A good way to do this is to add one extra serving of fruit, vegetable, oats products, beans, or peas each week.

Alcohol

Studies of people who drink one to two alcoholic beverages a day (12 oz. of beer, 4 oz. of wine, 1½ oz. of 80-proof [40 percent] alcohol) show a decreased rate in cardiac death. Death rates have been noted to be reduced in some studies by as much as 50 percent. About one-half of the benefit of the alcohol is attributed to an increase in HDL cholesterol and the remaining half of the benefit is the focus of ongoing studies—that is, we don't know yet! Beware, however, if the amount of alcohol consumption increases above two drinks a day: at this level you risk high blood pressure and an *increase* in heart disease and strokes. One good way to add alcohol to your diet is to have one glass of wine with lunch or dinner and/or one cordial in the evening.

The benefit of this dietary strategy is outweighed by its risk in people who are alcohol dependent. DO NOT start this regime if you have had trouble with overconsumption of alcohol in the past. Even with this modest amount of alcohol I pick a time and setting that will not require me to drive—and you should do the same!

Omega-3 fats

Omega-3 fats from fish oil and the vegetable form of omega-3, ALA from flaxseed or canola oil, should be part of every diet. The studies of Eskimos living in Greenland noted that a diet rich in cold-water fish was associated with a low incidence of heart attacks. Subsequent studies of different populations (including the Physician Health Study and the Nurses Health Study in the United States) showed that cardiovascular events were decreased when participants ate one to two fish meals a week. The results of the GISSI study in Italy showed that cardiac patients taking fish oil capsules every day had a lower incidence of sudden cardiac death compared to patients on a placebo capsule or a vitamin capsule. This cardioprotective effect is attributed to two unique fatty acids that are found in fish and fish oil, EPA and DHA. Because of the increasing concentration of mercury and PCPs in fish, both ocean- and fresh-water, as noted above, limited fish consumption is advised. Instead, focus on obtaining most of your omega-3 fatty acids from fish oil capsules (from major producers who state on the label that testing found the product to be free of mercury contamination). Another alternative is synthetic DHA made by processing ocean plant materials—no fish are involved. This form of DHA is free of mercury and other contaminants.

Soy Proteins

A review of studies of the consumption of soy proteins as part of a daily diet has shown that eating an average of 47 grams of soy protein a day resulted in a drop in LDL cholesterol of about 9 percent and a reduction in triglycerides of 11 percent, without a change in HDL cholesterol. The precise active ingredients in soy protein that lower cholesterol are still being studied, but the most likely substances are the isoflavones. These are powerful antioxidants whose benefits in preventing atherosclerosis have been described.

DETERMINING A HEART-HEALTHY WEIGHT

Study upon study has shown that being overweight increases your chances of developing heart disease. Obesity is a risk factor of particular concern to women, in part because being mildly overweight is associated with a more significant increase in cardiovascular risk for women than for men.

Of additional concern is the distribution of body fat in some overweight men and women. The risk of developing heart disease increases to a greater degree when the fat is located in the abdomen (measured by the ratio in inches of the waist to the hips), than when it is mostly located in the hips, thighs, and arms. The New Rules strategy for women is to measure your height and weight and calculate your BMI, and then measure your waist as well. If your BMI is over 25, and more so if it is over 29, or if your waist measurement is greater than 35 inches in women and 40 inches in men, a diet and exercise program is not just a good idea—it's a New Rules necessity!

Obesity in anyone, but particularly in women, is, in a sense, an emergency waiting to happen, and should be addressed as such by you and your doctor.

To determine your body weight relative to a healthy body weight, calculate your BMI and compare it to the recommended values.

How to Figure Your BMI

First, weigh yourself (use a balance or electrically calibrated scale) and measure your height with the movable measure on the balance scale or a wall-mounted height scale. BMI is calculated as your weight in kilograms, divided by the square of your height in meters. For those of us who aren't familiar with metric units, BMI can be looked up on the tables in Appendix I using inches and pounds, or it can be closely approximated with the following formula, which also uses inches and pounds. Next, using a cloth tape, measure the largest part of your abdomen: this may or may not be your waist. Do this standing and without any restrictive garments. The tape measure at your waist should be slightly firm but not tight enough to compress the waist.

$$\text{BMI} = (\text{Weight in pounds}/\text{Height in inches})^2 \times 703$$

Now calculate your heart-disease risk if you are overweight or obese by finding where your BMI fits in the table in Appendix II. Look at your classification with regard to obesity, and and then compare the numbers to the following table from the National Institutes of Health's Clinical Guideline on Obesity. If you are above the normal body weight range (BMI over 30), look up your risk in one of the two waist size columns on the upper right-hand side of the chart (see Appendix II).

If your BMI is under 25, you do not have a weight issue and can continue your current calorie intake unless you have to restrict your activity for any significant length of time, for instance, if you were to break your leg. In this case you should reduce calories by 200 to 500 calories a day from the carbohydrate and fat components of your dieting.

As you go up from 25, your risk for developing cardiovascular disease increases. With a BMI of 30, it is significant and more so if you have central obesity (a pear shape), as determined by a waist measurement of greater than 40 inches in a man and 35 inches in a women. In this case, your diet and activity pattern should be adjusted to lose one to two pounds a week until your

BMI is reduced to 25 or less. This means dropping your daily calorie intake by 500 calories a day. The National Institutes of Health weight loss guidelines suggest a six-month commitment to this program, after which you would expect to see a weight loss of 12 to 24 pounds.

If you are significantly overweight (obese or extremely obese), losing weight and keeping it off is a big challenge. Most of us know from our own experience that most diet programs fail; many are associated with weight gain, and even successful diets are usually followed by regaining of the weight lost (and often more) within six months. Regaining weight happens not only to you or some people; it is the finding in an overwhelming majority of studies. The NIH guidelines noted that the first goal of a weight loss program is to prevent further weight gain! An increase in exercise has, surprisingly, *not* been shown in studies to increase weight loss by itself. It has, however, been strongly associated with maintaining your weight at the new reduced level and should be increased to a minimum of 30 minutes of moderate activity a day when starting the program.

A very well-designed but "sobering" study done at Tufts–New England Medical Center and published in the *Journal of the American Medical Association* in 2005 studied patient outcome during the year after patients received motivational and instructional sessions regarding four popular diets: the Atkins diet (very low carbohydrate, high fat); the Ornish diet (very low fat, high carbohydrate); the Zone diet (intermediate levels of fat and carbohydrate); and the Weight Watchers diet, a balanced program in which points are assigned to different food groups. Researchers found that at one year, only 50 to 60 percent of patients described themselves as adhering to the diet. Weight loss and reduction in LDL cholesterol were similar for all the subjects in this study. What researchers learned from this study was that adherence to a

OBESITY IN WOMEN

The Nurses Health Study showed that women who were overweight with a BMI of between 25 and 29 had almost twice the risk of cardiovascular disease events when compared with women at or below ideal weight (BMI less than 25). To put this in terms perhaps easier to understand, if you are a five-foot, four-inch-tall woman, you should weigh 140 pounds or less to have a BMI below 25 and to not have a weight-related increase in heart attack risk. You would need to be below 155 pounds to avoid the important increased risk of being overweight at a BMI of 27 or more. At 175 pounds, a five-foot, four-inch woman would have a BMI of 30 and be classified as obese, with a dramatic increase in risk for developing diabetes, high blood pressure, and the metabolic syndrome that all contribute to a very high risk of heart disease and stroke.

For the one-in-four women aged 35 to 64 who are obese (BMI greater than 29), the risk of developing cardiovascular disease is increased more than threefold! An analysis of the women in the 26-year follow-up report of the Framingham study determined that 30 percent of the cardiovascular disease in these women is due to their obesity. (This is a big number and significantly more important than in men.)

diet with appropriate caloric intake was the important factor in losing weight, not the specifics of the diet. This is, in part, behind my selection of a modified DASH diet, since in my experience, patients find it an "easy" and tasty diet to stick with.

CONSULT A REGISTERED DIETICIAN

My clear first choice of how to begin a heart-healthy and, if required, weight-loss, diet is to set up an appointment with a registered dietician (RD) who will help you modify your diet and reduce your daily calories. The RD is also trained to help you develop behavior skills to remain focused and motivated throughout this process. Follow-up meetings can address your barriers to diet adherence and help you develop strategies to overcome these barriers. I had just such a meeting with a valued colleague and friend who is an RD before I started to write this chapter. This is a very important issue if your BMI is high, and if your odds of success in losing weight on your own are small. You need to do everything possible to increase your chances of success, and the cost of a consultation and follow-up with an RD is frequently covered by your medical plan. Ask your doctor to refer you. Even if the fee is not covered, a meeting with an RD is, to my thinking, money well spent.

UNDERSTAND THE MIND-BODY CONNECTION: GETTING A GRIP ON DEPRESSION, ANXIETY, AND STRESS CAN SAVE YOUR LIFE!

We've all experienced a fast pulse, palpitations, or a more forceful heartbeat that can accompany excitement, anger, or stress, and are therefore aware of some relationship between our minds and our hearts. These physical reactions are the results of impulses that originate in the brain and travel down to the heart. The concept that our thoughts, feelings, and reactions might affect the development of atherosclerosis in the coronary arteries, elevate our blood pressure, or provoke sudden death from a heart arrhythmia is, however, a relatively recent one. Understanding the connection—and modifying our behavior—is an important New Rules strategy for outliving heart disease.

This chapter reviews the science behind the linking of our state of mind to our heart disease. The issues for each of us are, of course:

- Does this link apply to me?
- Do I have these negative emotions (most of us do to some extent) that might raise my risk of heart disease?
- If so, what can I do about it?

Asking yourself some of the general questions that I present, and then answering the short list of more specific questions (the New Rules–Mind-Body Questions Scale) is a good start. I then present the strategies that I have found to be the most effective in combating these negative emotions. The goal here is to make our feelings and our energy work for us—not against us!

THE SCIENTIFIC FINDINGS

What we think and how we feel play a big role in the development of heart disease. How do we know about this mind-body connection to the condition of our hearts? Is it possible to measure or quantify this elusive concept? Many studies have done just that, with sometimes astounding results that impact our ability to outlive heart disease.

The first real observation of the mind-body connections that impact coronary disease was made by a cardiologist and a psychologist (Drs. Meyer Friedman and Ray Rosenman) in California. They shared an office and noted a personality type that was common among Dr. Friedman's heart patients. The patients who came in to see Dr. Friedman, the cardiologist, were more likely to be competitive, driven, concerned about time and how much they could achieve. They spoke quickly and were prone to finish others' sentences. They became very upset and agitated with delays. Drs. Friedman and Rosenman termed this combination of characteristics the Type A behavior pattern. They diagnosed this pattern using a scripted videotaped interview during which the interviewer recorded and scored speech and body motion characteristics that reflected time urgency and hostility.

Friedman and Rosenman's early work was the basis of a large epidemiological study, named the Western Collaborative Study (published in 1975) of over 3,000 men who did not have heart disease at the start of the study. At the end of the study eight and a half years later, they found that Type A men had twice the chance of developing a manifestation of coronary disease than those without Type A personality (called Type B). A subsequent study (published in 1980) using the people in the Framingham Study, including women, found a similar increase in heart disease with Type A personality. This statistical relationship of the Type A behavior pattern to heart disease was an independent risk factor, with about the same importance as an elevated cholesterol level or blood pressure reading. On the basis of this study and others, the Type A coronary event–prone behavior pattern became recognized as a risk factor for coronary heart disease, thus beginning the exploration of the relationship of the mind to heart disease.

Follow-up studies of the Type A behavior pattern noted that the hostility component was the most predictive of coronary heart disease. When a large nationwide study of heart disease risk factors, the Multiple Risk Factor Intervention Trial (MRFIT, published in 1985), found that measurements of a person's hostility, not their behavioral type, were predictive of future contrary events, the focus on Type A behavior shifted to other characteristics, including the following.

Hostility

As a personality trait, hostility is characterized by cynical beliefs, mistrust, and a display of anger and aggression when faced with problems. When this emotion was measured with a questionnaire in 424 patients undergoing coronary angiography, it was a significant predictor in men and women for the presence of contrary artery disease. A high hostility score increased the patient's likelihood of a positive angiogram more than threefold! Another compelling study looked at 255 physicians who had completed a hostility questionnaire while they were students at the North Carolina School of Medicine. Twenty-five years later, the students with the highest hostility scores were almost five times more likely to have had a heart attack, and nearly seven times more likely to have died!

Anger

Anger and hostility were initially thought to be the same emotion, but recent studies suggest that they are distinct and pose distinct risk factors. Anger is scored as a "trait" (a person commonly feels angry) or as a "state" (how angry a person feels at a given moment). Trait scores have been significantly predictive of heart disease in population studies, and therefore meet the criteria of a risk factor. Anger that is felt but not expressed is called "anger-in"; anger that is expressed is "anger-out." Studies show that if you routinely experience anger-in, you are at increased risk of cardiac events and high blood pressure when compared with people who express their anger. In contrast to these findings are those of the Myocardial Infarction Onset study (described in detail in the New Rule No. 4 on exercise), in which heart attack patients were questioned about the events just prior to their heart attacks; the results showed the danger of expressed angry moments (anger-out) in triggering a coronary event. Angry events—those likely to produce a surging heart rate and elevated blood pressure—were more than twice as likely to have occurred in the two hours before a heart attack than at other times.

Anxiety

Studies that have looked at anxiety levels and panic in both healthy people and patients with heart disease have shown that these emotions, too, predict heart events in a statistically important manner. A study of nearly 40,000 male health professionals called the Normative Aging Study (published in 1994) noted that in the two years following the completion of a brief psychosocial questionnaire, the findings of a high score for phobic anxiety was associated with a sixfold increase in the risk of sudden death.

Depression

The association of depression and coronary heart disease is remarkable to those of us who have studied such predictors. It's well known that people who have coronary events become depressed. This connection seems logical, but large-scale studies have now confirmed that depression is a powerful *predictor* of the future development of coronary disease in healthy people, as well as of cardiac events and death in patients who already have heart disease. When depressed individuals were compared to those who were not depressed, depression predicted the future development of coronary heart disease in a comparable manner to high blood pressure or cigarette smoking. One compelling study involved 1,190 medical students at Johns Hopkins University between 1948 and 1964. Each year they filled out a questionnaire that included a series of questions that were used to assess depression. In the male subjects with high depression questionnaire scores, the risk of a heart attack was twice as high as the nondepressed group, despite the presence of blood pressure, cholesterol, and cigarette smoking risk factors in both groups.

Depression is an even more powerful predictor of heart

Depression and Risk of MI Johns Hopkins Precursors Study

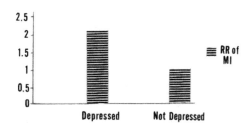

1,290 Male Students 40 Yrs. Follow-up of Depression and MI

attacks and survival in patients with heart disease. This is true even after the extent of heart disease measured as the damage to heart muscle or the level of cardiac symptoms is taken into consideration. These studies measured what is termed major depression, a significant clinical finding. In 1993, Drs. François Lesperance and Nancy Frasure-Smith at the Montreal Heart Institute published the results of a study in which they interviewed 430 patients who had survived heart attacks and correlated their survival rates at one year after the interview. Even after the researchers statistically adjusted the death rates on the basis of the amount of heart damage, the depressed patients had a greater than fourfold increase in death or heart attack compared to the nondepressed patients.

Cumulative Post–MI Mortality for Depressed and Nondepressed Patients

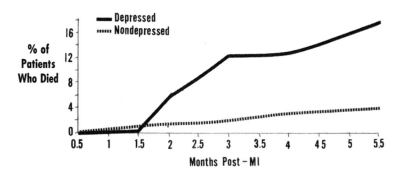

Of even greater importance to most of us are the studies that show a poorer prognosis in cardiac patients with only a depressed mood, termed minor depression. Minor depression is a very common finding in healthy men and women as well as those who already have heart disease. Dr. J. Barefoot and his colleagues at Duke University in 1996 used a questionnaire to assess depression in more than 1,000 patients with heart disease. They found that moderate to severely depressed patients were at about 85 percent greater risk than nondepressed patients of having a heart event over a long follow-up period (up to 19 years) and that mild depression increased risk by about 50 percent as compared to nondepressed patients.

In Canada, clinical scientists, also in 1996, looked at the impact of a "bundle" of the cardiac-prone emotions—anxiety, anger, and depression—that they termed distress, and noted a greater predictive value of coronary heart disease than the detection and scoring of any one of the three emotions in the bundle. A subsequent study of Finnish men (published in 1998) scored the extent of the combination of anger, depression, and anxiety (as distress) and combined this score with an assessment of an individual's absence of social coping skills and resources to yield what they called a measurement of "Type D ('D' is for distressed) personality." The investigators noted a 4.7-fold increase in cardiac events in men with an elevated Type D score. The greater value of the bundled emotions and social characteristics as compared with a single measured emotion or characteristic indicates that the relationship is very real but also very complex.

Social Stress

Social stress and its antitheses, social support and social cohesiveness, are, as suggested in the Finnish study I described, powerful factors in the development or prevention of heart disease.

There are a number of studies that show this relationship, but one of the best examples of the role of social stress in heart disease is a study of male monkeys (published in 1987). Aggressive male monkeys are driven to establish their dominant role in any group. In this study monkeys were fed a diet high in fat and cholesterol and dominant males were either allowed to remain in their first group or were frequently switched to different groups so that they were repeatedly required to establish their dominant position. These "socially stressed" male monkeys were found, at the end of the study, to have twice the amount of coronary atherosclerosis as dominant males who were left in a stable setting.

MITIGATING FACTORS

Social Support

Having people you can confide in and the skills with which to confide in them is considered a buffer to the effects of coronary event–prone emotions. All of us encounter "stressors" in our daily life that can potentially stimulate anger, anxiety, and depression. Having a frame of reference in which to place the stressors and the ability and resources to discuss them with a family member or friend would mitigate the intensity of the emotional response and thus could protect us from coronary atherosclerosis. In a Finnish study (published in 1988) of 13,301 men and women without heart disease, social support was assessed as the sum of four types of social connections:

- Marriage
- Contacts with extended family or friends
- Church membership
- Other group associations

The investigators found that people with the lowest quarter of social support scores had twice the likelihood of dying as people with the highest scores in the highest quarter. Social support is a significant protective behavior that is thought to counteract, in part, effects of coronary-prone emotions on heart disease.

Social Cohesiveness

The support of a society and culture with comforting values and roles has also been demonstrated to have a powerful protective effect. An interesting example of this is the town of Roseto, Pennsylvania. In the 1950s this town was made almost entirely of people who had immigrated from Roseto, Italy; the population was close-knit, Roman Catholic, and patriarchal. It had an unusually low incidence of coronary death compared to a neighboring town, Bangor, despite nearly identical fat content in diet and a similar degree of obesity. Bangor, however, was a polyethnic town, with less emphasis on traditional family roles, and investigators postulated that the social cohesiveness of the transported traditional Italian village was cardioprotective. Over the following 25 years, the traditional values in Roseto gave way to the more diverse American standards, and the rate of heart disease rose to equal its neighboring town. Another study that looked at social cohesiveness involved nearly 4,000 Japanese Americans in San Francisco. The investigators compared the coronary heart disease rates among those who were brought up with an American lifestyle and those whose upbringing reflected strong ties to the traditional Japanese culture. The heart disease rate was 2.5 times less in those brought up in the traditional Japanese culture.

HOW CORONARY-PRONE EMOTIONS AND LOW SOCIAL SUPPORT IMPACT YOUR HEART

Although our understanding of the exact mechanisms of emotions as risk factors for heart disease is still very much a work in progress, there are several types of alterations in the body's normal biology and physiology that may explain, in part, the effect of the cardiac event–prone emotions on atherosclerosis and coronary events, such as angina and heart attacks.

The Autonomic, or "Involuntary," Nervous System

The first of these alterations is the balance of the sympathetic and parasympathetic nervous systems in a person at rest. As I indicated in the introduction to this chapter, the sympathetic nervous system is activated during periods of physical and psychological stress and results in an increase in heart rate from impulses that travel down the sympathetic nerves to the heart. In addition, the sympathetic nervous system acts on our adrenal glands (these are midway down our back, on the sides of our body right above our kidneys) to produce adrenaline in the bloodstream, which stimulates the heart muscles to contract more forcefully and dilates or constricts blood vessels in various parts of the body. The sympathetic system acts as part of the fight-or-flight response; we do not consciously control it.

In contrast, when we are relaxed, are not stressed or fearful, and physically at rest, the sympathetic system becomes much less active, and the predominant system is the parasympathetic, or vagel, nervous system, named after the major nerve in this system, the vagus nerve. Impulses from this system slow the heart, lower blood pressure, and increase the digestion.

The sympathetic system and its opposite-acting parasympathetic system are termed the autonomic, or involuntary, nervous system.

It was thought that the psychological state of arousal associated with anger and anxiety would lead to persistent activation of the sympathetic nervous system and a resulting increase in adrenaline in the blood, which would enhance atherosclerosis through damage to the vessels' endothelial cells. In the past several years we have developed a way to measure the balance of the two systems at rest. This measurement, called Heart Rate Variability, is done by looking at the very small differences in time between each heartbeat. Although our pulse usually feels perfectly regular, there are actually small variations in the intervals between the heartbeats. When these small variations are analyzed by a mathematical process called a Fast Fourier Transform, we can evaluate the relative impact of the sympathetic and the parasympathetic nervous systems on the heart. A high sympathetic and low parasympathetic component profile is a powerful predictor of future cardiovascular events and death in people with heart disease. Studies of patients with depression show these same high sympathetic and lower parasympathetic components, supporting the concept that depression alters the balance of the sympathetic to parasympathetic nervous systems to increase heart attack risk.

The Cerebral-Pituitary-Adrenal Axis

A second possible mechanism is an increase in the brain's signals to the pituitary gland to produce a messenger chemical that stimulates, in turn, our adrenal glands, which sit atop each of our kidneys and produce cortisol. This mechanism is called the cerebral-pituitary-adrenal axis, and is used every day by the brain to alter the biological system for day (active stress) and night (safe rest). This axis is also a critical part of the body's response to injury and stress, helping, among other things, to expand our blood volume and increase the activity of our platelets to form clots. All of these mechanisms are critical parts of the fight-or-flight response. When they occur occasionally over a brief time period (as in running from a tiger!) they are life-saving, but when this response occurs on an almost continuous daily basis, production of cortisol rises (elevated levels of cortisol are found in patients affected by depression) and will accelerate atherosclerosis and increase the risk of heart attacks.

Coronary Event–Prone Emotions

Another mechanism that seems to increase heart attack risk is not biological or physiological, but rather behavioral; that is, the coronary event–prone emotions lead to an increase of other coronary heart-disease risk factors. Angry, depressed, and anxious patients are more likely to be sedentary, eat a high-fat diet, smoke, and neglect to treat elevated blood pressure. In a study of heart attack patients who were prescribed a single aspirin pill a day, being depressed resulted in a full 33 percent reduction in the likelihood that the patient would take the aspirin, which would have reduced the risk of a second heart attack by almost 25 percent!

A NEW RULES STRATEGY TO DETERMINE MIND-BODY RISK FACTORS THAT COULD AFFECT YOUR HEART

How can you transform the information gleaned from these studies into a New Rules strategy to prevent heart disease, or to prevent coronary events if you already have it?

Step I: Decide if these emotions and social structure describe you.

Look at and listen to your body motions, your words, actions, and feelings, and then ask yourself if you experience any of these emotions—anger, anxiety, or depression—*on a daily basis*. In a paper on psychological risk factors and heart disease published in the *American Journal of Cardiology* in 2005, Dr. Alan Rozanski and colleagues suggested five questions that a cardiologist should ask his or her patients regarding these factors. I think they are very good questions to ask ourselves as we try to determine if these issues are important for us and so I have paraphrased them in that context as follows:

1. Would you characterize yourself as having a low energy level, that is, are you frequently tired or listless?
2. Do you have restful sleep or are you having trouble sleeping and awake feeling unrefreshed?
3. Is your mood upbeat or are you feeling blue, depressed, sad, or angry on more than a rare occasion?
4. Do you feel under a lot of pressure or stress at work or at home?
5. Do you have a family member or a friend whom you can confide in, with whom you can discuss your problems, and who cares about your feelings?

If any of these questions "ring a bell" for you, then you will find real value in addressing these issues. The more complete set of New Rules–Mind-Body Questions that follow are selected from a variety of questionnaires that I have used to help patients assess their "mind risk factors." If you are uncertain as to whether to pursue these issues, reading and thinking about these questions may help. My threshold for using the techniques that I discuss at the end of this chapter is very low, since there is almost no downside. In other words, if you answer yes to even one of these questions, you might want to think about getting some additional assistance to address the issue. The worst that can happen is that you will become more in touch with your feelings and, one would hope, become a happier person.

Step 2: Fill Out the New Rules–Mind-Body Questions Scale

Below are questions regarding six coronary-relevant emotions and your level of social support.

1. Anger

   Do you often feel angry or irritated?

   Do you frequently feel like shouting, throwing things, or using curse words?

   Does your anger interfere with your relationships at home or at work?

2. Anxiety

   Do you often feel anxious?

   Do you often find that you are jittery or jumpy?

   Do you regularly worry that something bad could happen?

   Would you describe yourself as under tension on a daily basis?

3. Depression

   The following are the criteria for depression. If you experience five of these criteria, there is a reasonable likelihood you are significantly depressed.

_____Depressed mood

_____Reduced interest or pleasure in activities

_____Weight loss or gain of over 5 percent of your usual weight, a decrease in appetite, or sleep problems

_____Nervous agitation

_____Feelings of worthlessness or excessive guilt

_____Difficulty concentrating

_____Repeated thoughts of death or of committing suicide

Some questions to ask yourself include:

Do you feel sad or unworthy some of the time, or more frequently?

Do you cry or feel like crying some of the time, or more frequently?

Are you unable to sleep well and/or do you have trouble getting going in the morning?

4. Social Support [Answer yes or no.]

Is there a special person around when you need someone?

Do you get the emotional help and support you need from your family?

Is there a special person who really cares about your feelings?

Do you talk about your problems with friends?

5. Hostility [True or false?]

I often have to take orders from someone who does not know as much as I do.

I require a lot of argument to convince most people of
  the truth.
I think most people would lie to get ahead.
Most people inwardly dislike putting themselves out to
  help other people.

6. General Distress [Answer yes or no.]
  Do you frequently complain of headaches?
  Are you annoyed or irritated easily?
  Do you often feel down or blue?
  Do you frequently feel fearful or worried?
  Are you often self-conscious or uncomfortable around
    other people?

If your answer is yes to some of these questions, you most
likely do have, as do many of us, psychosocial, or "mind," risk
factors for coronary heart disease. Addressing these risk factors
is a critically important aspect of outliving heart disease by the
New Rules, and of perhaps equal or more importance in enhancing the enjoyment of our lives. For strategies on how to address
these factors, read on!

THE NEW RULES STRATEGY TO ADDRESS MIND-BODY RISK FACTORS FOR DEVELOPING HEART DISEASE

If you have determined that you are at risk for developing heart
disease or for not outliving your heart disease due to mind-body
risk factors, there are several New Rules–recommended
approaches that you should try.

Individual Therapy

The clear first choice in dealing with mind-body risk factors is to get an expert opinion and professional assistance, if this is available, affordable, and something you are comfortable doing. A psychiatrist or psychologist is the best-trained professional in this regard, and one or two sessions should detect and assess coronary event–prone risk emotions, personality traits, and social behaviors. This process will often involve completing a questionnaire or group of short questionnaires that may include some of the New Rules–Mind-Body Questions, the scores from which will provide you and the psychologist with important information.

If you are aware from your feelings or through feedback from those around you that you are continually or frequently depressed; easily angered; often worried and anxious about different things; and feel alone, with no one in whom to confide, it is essential that you contact a psychiatrist or psychologist. Ask your physician for a recommendation. These consultations may well be one of the most important of your strategies to outlive heart disease!

Remember that there are now very effective medications to treat depression, anxiety, and panic disorder. These drugs can make a real difference in your feelings and behavior, but you'll need to be under the care of a psychiatrist, who will prescribe them and monitor their effects on you.

Group Therapy

Another excellent option, if it is available in your area, is a group program, usually run by a psychologist, especially for patients with coronary heart disease or with high cardiac risk emotional personality or social factors. I have been impressed with the value of one such group therapy program led by a cardiac-trained psychologist, Dr. Robert Allen. For more than 10 years this group was part of the Coronary Intervention and Prevention Program, which I helped to start in 1975 and now codirect at the 92nd Street Y in New York City. These mind factors are not only important because of the cardiac risk, but because they negatively impact our lives and our ability to enjoy living. For many of my patients, joining this group or other similar programs was a wonderful gift that they gave themselves.

Self-help groups run by trained nurses, exercise physiologists, or nutritionists can often be of help. The focus of the group, its members, and the leader's skill and experience are critical factors in the value of this approach. One of the most successful studies of emotional, nutritional, and exercise intervention in heart disease patients, the Ornish study cited group sessions with specially trained leaders as a critical component of its success.

OTHER OPTIONS

Finally, there are a number of other effective things that you can do for yourself to deal with mind-body risk factors.

Exercise

Start a regular exercise program, such as the one described in New Rule No. 4. Exercise has been especially effective in treating mild depression. You should exercise every day or at least three times a week, at least a half hour per session, and include dynamic low-resistance exercises like walking, jogging, cycling, swimming, dance calisthenics, or use rowing, stepping, or elliptical exercise machines. Your best choice is to join a class or work out in a place with others, thereby getting social support at the same time. Joining a gym works especially well for men, who seem to interact better in athletic settings than in other settings. But don't hesitate! If joining a gym is a barrier to beginning your exercise routine, just start a walking program on your own. See the chapter on exercise beginning on page 73 for more details.

Read *The Feeling Good Handbook*

Read and work through *The Feeling Good Handbook* by Dr. David Burns. This is a cognitive therapy workbook that has been highly effective at helping people understand their emotions. It consciously helps them to feel better, and thus live longer. For people who can use books of this nature, and we should all try, it is very effective.

Be an Active Listener

Re-establish contacts with family and friends and work on being an active listener. Active listening is attentive listening without interruption, but with responses that show you are involved in the discussion. Good eye contact and a relaxed posture also help. Few things are as engaging as active listening. You will find you enjoy this, are responded to in kind, and are building a socially supportive connection with friends and family members.

Engage in the Meditative Arts

Try yoga, meditation, tai chi—anything that focuses your mind calms your body. The next chapter is devoted to complementary medicine that examines this phenomenon in more detail.

EXPLORE COMPLEMENTARY MEDICINES AND ALTERNATIVE TREATMENTS

If you are like most Americans, you use one or more alternative medical treatment and, when you see your doctor, forget to mention it! Population surveys have noted that more than two-thirds of Americans use or have used alternative therapies, including herbs and vitamin supplements, homeopathic remedies, and specific treatments not recognized to be of value by traditional Western clinical science. In patients who reported the use of these alternative therapies, one-half stated that they did not share this information with their physicians.

The high level of interest in and use of alternative therapies to prevent heart disease may reflect our desire for treatments that are "natural," and have in many instances been used for generations in our culture. It helps that these treatments are often less expensive than prescribed medications and that they provide a means of "empowering" us to take charge of our own health, as opposed to being "cared for" by a doctor.

While your New Rules program should include certain alternative therapies, such as some form of meditation or prayer, you need to be careful when choosing complementary medicines, in the form of herbal supplements and vitamins, to achieve your goal of outliving your heart disease.

This chapter does several things:

First, it explains the issues and procedures used to *establish the effectiveness* of traditional treatments for heart disease, and notes why some of these complementary medicines fall so short of these procedures that your doctor's enthusiasm for recommending them might be compromised—and why you should be wary before using them.

Second, it looks at certain *herbal and vitamin supplements* that have been used to treat heart disease symptoms and illuminates which ones work and which ones to avoid in a New Rules–approved treatment plan.

Finally, you'll learn of several *alternative therapies*—including meditation and prayer—that many patients have found useful in their New Rules program to outlive heart disease.

DETERMINING THE EFFECTIVENESS OF TRADITIONAL AND NONTRADITIONAL TREATMENTS

Whatever your motivation, the important issues surrounding alternative treatments and complementary medicines with regard to our New Rules program to outlive heart disease are:

1. Is the treatment effective (that is, Does it work?), and if so, how does its effectiveness compare with prescribed medical therapies?
2. Is the treatment dangerous by itself or when used in conjunction with standard medical care as a complementary therapy?
3. Is the treatment keeping you from an effective

preventive or treatment program and thus denying you
the benefit of proven therapies?

A good starting point to answer these questions is the concern
that physicians have with their use.

The first concern is the lack of oversight in the United States
in the preparation and sale of vitamins and other supplements.
In 1994 Congress passed, and President Clinton signed, legislation placing these products outside the purview of the Federal
Drug Administration, which requires clear evidence of efficacy
and safety before a pharmaceutical can be sold. Also, and often
of equal importance, the FDA can oversee the continued collection of data with regard to any adverse long-term effects of the
drug and any drug-drug interactions that could lead to patient
harm. On the other hand, supplements, including herbal preparations, vitamins, minerals, amino acids (the building blocks of
proteins), and oils may be produced without inspections or oversight by the FDA (or any agency for that matter). What this
means is that general claims can be made in ads or on the supplement's packaging label based on small studies that may not be
designed to rigorous scientific standards and that have not been
critically reviewed by the FDA. Only when there is evidence of
danger to people, most often from reports in the medical literature or the press (such as the article that appeared in the *Journal
of the American Medical Association* in 2004 noting high levels
of mercury contamination of some herbs imported from China)
can the FDA bring action to ban its sale. In essence, supplement
manufacturing is an unregulated industry that sells billions of
dollars in products for the treatment and prevention of disease.
Over the past several years there have been cases of patient illness and death from these products or the adulteration of the
product during production and packaging.

The second concern is that only a very few herbs or supplements have been studied with the large, controlled, and blinded clinical trials that are required of every new drug that the FDA approves for use. Thus, knowledge of the benefit and safety of the supplements is based on the perceptions of the practitioners who use these products and patients who feel the products have helped them. Making clinical decisions based on the quality of the evidence supporting how effective a treatment is in helping you and the likelihood of the treatment harming you is called evidence-based medicine. Evidence-based medicine is not only the basis of sound medical practice but also of each of the New Rules for outliving heart disease outlined in this book. The "gold standard" of such evidence are the outcomes of large clinical trials in which patients have been assigned, at random, to the treatment or, if possible, a placebo. In the case of a drug, herb, vitamin, or other supplement, the placebo would be a sugar pill.

Large, well-designed studies work because patients with unknown factors that might affect a drug's performance should end up equally in the treatment or the placebo group and therefore the unknown factor does not affect the outcome of the study. Also, in these studies the patients and the scientists caring for the patients and performing the tests are blinded with regard to whether a specific patient is receiving the product or a placebo, thus preventing their beliefs about the drug from tainting the data. Finally, these studies are prospective, meaning that the data is collected going forward in time after the patients are randomly assigned to treatment or placebo. This eliminates the factors that would affect outcome but cannot be appreciated when we collect the data by asking the patient to recall specific facts.

A faster and cheaper technique is called a case-cohort study, in which patients with a disease and healthy people of the same age are asked about their prior and current use of a treatment. A much higher rate of the treatment's use in healthy people compared with those who have the disease is strongly suggestive of the treatment's value. However, this kind of study can come to the wrong conclusion if all the factors that could confound the findings are not considered—and it is often impossible to do so. A relatively well-known example of a case-cohort study is the one that addressed the use of hormone replacement therapy in women. Early data from the Nurses Health Study, run by the epidemiologists at Harvard, noted that nurses who had heart attacks were less likely to have reported the use of hormone therapy when they started in the study 10 years before than were women who had not had a heart attack. This data was evidence in favor of hormone replacement therapy to prevent heart attacks in women, but these women, along with their physicians, chose hormone therapy, so other factors may have played a role in producing this data, since women who chose hormone therapy may have lived a healthier lifestyle to begin with. (For one thing, they saw their doctors at least once a year to get their prescriptions renewed!) Using statistical methods, the data was corrected for the major known risk factors of developing heart disease, and the use of hormone therapy was still significant— and millions of women across the United States were treated with hormone therapy as they reached menopause. It wasn't until 2001 that data from a large randomized, blinded, placebo-controlled prospective clinical trial showed that women who started estrogen and progesterone combination therapy were actually at *increased* risk for having a heart attack during the first two years of therapy. Thus the conclusion reached from this case-cohort analysis of the Nurses Study was wrong, and patients suffered.

Based on this recent experience, it is not surprising that careful physicians want large clinical trials showing safety and efficacy before they prescribe any drug. So, despite a long track record of apparent safety, therapies such as vitamin or herbal supplements that have not been studied by clinical trials may, in fact, be dangerous, and physicians regard such supplementation with some skepticism!

There is, however, another side to this issue of rigorous testing. The other side includes the fact that in many cases the active ingredient in common pharmaceuticals is derived from plants, and many common medications, such as aspirin for fever and pain, and digitalis for heart failure, were in fact originally used as herbal treatments. Another issue is the fact that we are not likely to see in the near future the kind of large clinical trials of alternative therapies that the FDA requires for drug approval because of the enormous cost involved. Large random, controlled, and blinded trials now cost more than $10 million and only make economic sense, in the private sector, if a pharmaceutical company receives patent protection on the drug and is in a position to make a profit if the clinical trial and other studies are successful. No one owns the herbs! Thus, even if a certain treatment could be proved effective, there is no way that the supplement manufacturer could patent it and earn back the cost of the trial. The National Institutes of Health has a division that addresses alternative and complementary therapies and is funding some trials that will finally, I believe, prove or disprove efficacy and safety in some, but certainly not all, commonly used supplements.

Another shared concern about the safety and efficacy of supplements is that, since their manufacture is unregulated, we can never be sure of getting the dosages that the label says we are, or, of equal importance, if the dosages of the active ingredients are the same from package to package of the same product from the same company! Some companies now standardize their herbs and supplements to a given active ingredient, but many do not. Lack of government agency policy to require and monitor standardization of supplements is a safety issue that most physicians take very seriously.

THE NEW RULES–APPROVED USE OF HERBAL AND VITAMIN SUPPLEMENTS

In this section, I review the evidence and rationale for the more widely used complementary medicines, including herbal supplements, neutrachemicals, and vitamins, aimed at treating and preventing heart disease, and make rational recommendations based on the best available evidence concerning their safety and effectiveness. Such recommendations will be one of the following:

1. *Consider using:* There is some good evidence for efficacy and no issues of safety.
2. *Can use but not recommended:* The product is unlikely to help (or there is weak evidence of efficacy) but no issues of safety.
3. *Don't use:* There are issues of safety or there is no appropriate evidence of safety when used alone or in combination with other treatments.

Below is a list of the most popular complementary medicines for heart disease and what we need to know about them.

Herbal Supplements

Herbal supplements are derived from plants, but, as with other supplements, standardization in the manufacturing of these products is variable depending on the manufacturer, so you can never be sure if you are getting the proper amounts of the active ingredients to achieve the results you want. Part of the reason, I suspect, for their widespread use today is that these plant products have been used for generations to treat various ailments, and are thought of as more "natural" to take than prescription medications. Below is a list of the more common supplements used in the treatment of heart disease.

Artichoke (Cynara scolymus)

Recent studies have demonstrated that the extract of the artichoke leaf has a lipid-lowering effect presumed to be from the substance luteolin, which may inhibit co-A reductase activity in a similar fashion to the statins. A recent small clinical trial of short duration (five weeks) showed a significant reduction in cholesterol levels in the group that took dried artichoke extract compared to the control group. The only known potential adverse effect would be in patients with bile duct obstruction, as there is some speculation that artichokes may increase the flow of bile from the liver to the gall bladder.

Recommendation: This is a potentially interesting product that may have a role in reducing LDL and total cholesterol, but the studies proving that claim are very limited. Statins, which have been studied in large clinical trials for more than 10 years, achieve the same effect and have been proven safe for long-term usage. Pending further studies of artichoke leaf supplementation, I would recommend that my patients to enjoy artichokes with their food, but if they have elevated LDL, to take a physician-prescribed medication, such as a statin, to lower their reading.

Bishop's weed (Ammi visnaga)

Bishop's weed is used for the treatment of mild angina pectoris, and is so approved by the German Commission E (the German national organization that provides medical recommendation regarding the use of herbs and other supplements). It is postulated that it dilates coronary arteries due to two chemicals: visnagin and khellin. Clinical effectiveness of using this supplement is modest and nausea and headache are not uncommon side effects.

Recommendation: Because of its mild beneficial effect and

common disagreeable side effects, I would recommend avoiding use of this herb.

Garlic (Allium sativum)

Perhaps the most widely used herb for the treatment and prevention of heart disease, garlic has been noted in some small- to moderate-sized studies to be effective in lowering cholesterol and blood pressure, and inhibiting the formation of blood clots. It can be used raw, or cooked in food preparation, or taken as a supplement in the form of an oil or a tablet. The oil and tablet forms are usually standardized to allicin potential, which means that they have a defined concentration of the specific chemical (in this case, allicin) thought to be responsible for the pharmacological effects of the plant.

A recent analysis of multiple placebo-controlled studies using various preparations of garlic noted a reduction in LDL cholesterol, thought to be due to a mechanism similar to that of the statins. One such study noted a statistically significant reduction in LDL and total cholesterol at three months, but failed to find a significant reduction at six months. Another study of garlic powder supplementation demonstrated a reduction in blood pressure over a four-year period, but other studies have failed to confirm this finding. A review of published studies by the United States Department of Health's Agency for Health Care Research and Quality concluded that there was no evidence of a beneficial effect on blood pressure. Garlic supplementation has also been noted in selected studies to reduce platelet activation, a key element in forming a blood clot, and one intriguing study showed a reduction in measurement of carotid intimal medial thickness (this is a measurement of atherosclerosis in the main artery to the brain—see New Rule No. 8) in a group of patients receiving garlic pills when compared to progression shown in the placebo group.

One reason postulated for the differing study outcomes is the wide variation in allicin release from garlic supplements standardized to the same allicin content. Many of the products released less than 20 percent of the stated allicin content. These kinds of wide variations in a supplement's efficacy also raise safety issues. For example, given the potential of garlic to inhibit blood clots, garlic supplementation should be not be used by patients taking Coumadin because of the potential for enhanced risk of bleeding. Another example of the danger of using garlic was indicated in the beginning of this chapter: you might forget to tell your doctor you are taking it and, if you needed surgery, your blood clotting ability could be impaired, placing you at unnecessary risk.

Recommendation: Treatment of dyslipidemia and hypertension to guideline goals is too important to leave to a product not proven to be consistently effective. The long-term efficacy and safely of statins, blood pressure medications, and low-dose aspirin are clearly better choices. Garlic should be consumed as part of a healthy diet, but not, at present, as a supplement. For patients who do use garlic supplements, remember to stop one month before any elective surgery and do not use the supplements with drugs that affect clotting, such as Coumadin.

Ginkgo (Ginkgo biloba)

This widely used herb has been demonstrated to enhance dilatation of small arteries and, in small controlled studies, to reduce claudication, the muscle pain during walking that is due to disease of the arteries to the leg muscles. The German Commission E notes only occasional gastrointestinal upset, headache, and allergic skin reactions as side effects. There are a few reports of bleeding when gingko is given with drugs that are anticoagulants.

Recommendation: Efficacy is not proven, but risk, if you are not using Coumadin or aspirin, is reported as very low. As with garlic, do not use ginkgo with Coumadin, and stop this product one month before an anticipated surgery.

Guggul

Guggul is the product of a tree native to India, Pakistan, and Afghanistan, where it is used by practitioners as a treatment for elevated cholesterol, obesity, and joint pains. While small studies have demonstrated a modest reduction in total and LDL cholesterol, there are no well-performed clinical trials. Reported side effects include nausea and headache; contraindications include pregnancy.

Recommendation: This is an interesting product, but in the absence of well-performed clinical trials, not a prudent therapeutic choice.

Hawthorn (Crataegus oxyacantha)

Hawthorn is a fruit currently being studied as a treatment for cardiovascular disease, specifically congestive heart failure due to dysfunction of the heart wall muscle. Some reports indicate positive effects in the treatment of high blood pressure, angina, and elevated cholesterol levels. The German Commission E recognizes hawthorn for the treatment of mild congestive heart failure. Hawthorn is considered to be safe, with few reported side effects and wide usage.

Recommendation: At present, hawthorn provides, at best, limited efficacy for very early congestive heart failure. Recent studies have shown that aggressive treatment of early congestive heart failure can be of significant clinical value. The use of hawthorn in patients treated with medications including ACE inhibitors and beta-blockers has not been well studied. I would defer the use of hawthorn pending further studies.

Horse Chestnut (Aesculus hippocastanun)

Horse Chestnut is used as an extract of the seed and bark of the horse chestnut tree for chronic venous insufficiency, such as the enlargement of leg veins that causes leg swelling. There is a low incidence of side effects in the European literature (horse chestnut being widely used in Europe), but concerns exist regarding horse chestnut's anticoagulant effect. It is not used in patients taking Coumadin or other anticoagulants.

Recommendation: Except for its possible combination anticoagulation effects, there are no clear concerns regarding safety, but in the absence of large controlled trials of this substance, safety remains an issue. One recent review of the published data concluded that horse chestnut seed extract is an effective therapy for swollen veins in the leg.

Red Yeast Rice

This product, a dried powder prepared from fermentated white rice with the yeast *monascus purpureus*, contains statins, specifically lovastatin (Mevacor) in small amounts, as well as other ingredients. Several small clinical trials have noted significant reductions in total and LDL cholesterol and triglycerides, and most recently, a reduction in markers of inflammation and improvement in endothelial function—the same effects that have been noted with statins. A concern exists regarding the variation in quality and content of the available products. There are two major preparations of red yeast rice: cholestin and xuezhikang. Cholestin is prepared by the fermentation of a specific strain of the yeast to produce lovastatin (Mevacor). Xuezhikang is processed from rice and red yeast that have been mixed with alcohol. At the present time, these supplements are not sold in the United States because the FDA successfully sued in civil court by proving that the manufacturer was essentially selling lovastatin, a patented drug. Large studies regarding side effects and adverse effects are not available.

Recommendation: Given the enormous data on the safety and efficacy of the statins produced by the drug companies, it is not prudent to address high cholesterol levels with a statin produced by fermenting rice and yeast in an essentially unregulated manufacturing process. Such products vary in content and potency and lack the important clinical trials to determine their safety.

Neutrachemicals

Neutrachemicals are supplements that are neither herbs nor vitamins. They can be minerals or by-products of biological functions that have been isolated and found to have some effect, real or imagined, on a medical ailment. The same caution about lack of testing and standardization in the manufacture of these products, discussed earlier with regard to herbal supplements, applies to neutrachemicals.

Carnitine

When heart muscle is ischemic, that is, deprived of oxygen caused by reduced blood flow to the muscle itself, the concentration of carnitine decreases. Carnitine is a proteinlike substance important for its role in transporting fatty acids to the heart muscle, where it is converted into energy. It is postulated that increasing muscle carnitine levels with oral supplementation may reduce the impact of ischemia on the heart muscle. Several small studies showed inconsistent results (some show efficacy, some do not) when carnitine supplementation was given to patients with acute myocardial infarction. Carnitine deficiency is known to cause weakness in heart muscle and in the skeletal muscles of our body, and in some studies, carnitine supplementation has resulted in improvement in heart and skeletal muscles. One trial of 40 patients noted that carnitine was effective with regard to increasing heart muscle, but for unknown reasons was also associated with an increased rate of death and hospitalization.

Recommendation: Carnitine should be studied further with regard to efficacy and risk. At the moment, given the increased death rate in one trial of heart failure patients taking this supplement, carnitine should not be used.

Coenzyme Q$_{10}$

Also known as CoQ, this substance was identified in 1957 and is known to play an important role in the final stages of the metabolism of fats and sugars to produce energy. This process takes places in small structures in our cells called mitochondria. The product, available as a supplement, is produced from tobacco leaf, sugarcane, or beets, and is widely used in Japan, Russia, and Europe for the treatment of congestive heart failure and for its purported effects on blood pressure and angina pectoris. Several reasonably large and long-term studies that were not controlled (that is, they had no placebo arm of the study) noted improvement in heart muscle function, a lowering of elevated blood pressure, and increased exercise tolerance in angina pectoris. In contrast, several controlled studies have not shown a beneficial effect of CoQ on heart wall muscle in patients with congestive heart failure. There were no reported adverse events due to CoQ in a six-year study of subjects who used 100mg a day.

Recommendation: Despite some interesting positive results in studies of subjects who took CoQ and the positive reports of trials that did not have a placebo arm for comparison, the negative outcome from the small clinical trials is troublesome and I would not recommend use of this product until the results of larger trials that substantiate a value to the use of CoQ supplementation are available. There are no issues of safety according to published medical articles.

Creatine

This amino acid plays a role in the storage and regeneration of energy in muscle cells. It has been postulated that increased consumption of creatine will raise the levels in the muscles of our body and increase their strength. In a small trial creatine was given to patients with reduced exercise tolerance and was associated with an increase in the patients' ability to perform exercise. Adverse events that have been reported with use of creatine include nausea, fatigue, seizures, and general muscle weakness.

Recommendation: This supplement is popular among athletes, but studies have been inconsistent with regard to performance enhancement. Given the reported adverse events, it should only be used with your physician's knowledge, so that the symptoms, if they occur, are not misinterpreted. In most instances I would wait for further studies and knowledge about the effect of carnitine supplementation.

L-arginine

This is a supplement born from the scientific studies that demonstrated the role of the endothelial cells (the inner layer of the artery) in the dilation of the artery by the production of nitric oxide (NO). To produce NO, the endothelial cell metabolizes L-arginine. It is postulated that increasing L-arginine in the endothelial cells will enhance the production of NO. The importance of enhancing NO production goes beyond vasodilatation. Endothelial cells that fail to produce sufficient NO are termed dysfunctional and promote several critical steps in the development of the atherosclerotic plaques, whereas "functional" endothelial cells inhibit this process.

Studies of L-arginine supplementation include well-run small clinical trials that have, in all but two studies, shown clinical benefit in patients with coronary artery disease and angina pectoris, peripheral artery disease with leg pain while walking (claudication), and congestive heart failure. Studies in hypertensive patients failed to show a benefit. Reported side effects have included nausea and diarrhea. An impressive study using rabbits showed that L-arginine added to a high cholesterol diet inhibited the development of atherosclerosis. This result was not seen in the control group of rabbits.

Recommendation: This is a potentially important product in the treatment and prevention of atherosclerotic coronary artery disease. It would be utilized in patients on a variety of medications and thus contraindications need to be fully studied before it can be safely prescribed. L-arginine should be treated as a pharmaceutical, not a supplement, and its clinical use awaits further studies to define its effect and long-term safety. Even though its consumption by the public is currently not regulated—it is one ingredient in a product called a "Heart Bar"—it should not, in my opinion, be used as a supplement.

Selenium

This mineral, when deficient, is the cause of heart muscle weakness that can be fatal. However, selenium deficiency only occurs in certain regions of Asia.

Recommendation: Do not take selenium supplements.

Taurine

This is an amino acid that is found in high concentration in the heart muscle. Taurine deficiency is a rare cause of heart muscle disease that can be fully corrected by taurine supplementation. This use has focused attention on taurine as a possible supplement to enhance heart muscle function in congestive heart failure. Several small clinical trials (having fewer than 50 subjects in total) have shown improvement in heart muscle function in patients with congestive heart failure. Further studies are required to support these early findings and to learn about the interaction of taurine with the pharmaceuticals commonly prescribed to treat congestive heart failure and to determine its long-term effect on patient survival.

Recommendation: This is a very interesting supplement that shows promise in very small short-term trials. We are, however, not yet at the point where we know enough regarding taurine supplementation to recommend it to patients as a supplement. It is worth talking with your physician about this substance. Ask him or her to read about it if you are suffering from congestive heart failure.

Vitamins

Four out of 10 Americans take vitamins, most commonly a single multivitamin and mineral pill, every day. These pills usually contain one or more times the FDA's recommended daily allowance (RDA). When vitamins are consumed with the goal of preventing or treating heart disease, however, the doses are well above this range, often 10 to 100 times the RDA necessary to prevent a vitamin deficiency, and are used for their presumed antioxidant effect, which is to reduce the first minimal oxidation of LDL cholesterol in the intima layer of the arteries. This oxidation, if left unchecked, sets in motion the process of inflammation that characterizes progressive atherosclerosis. This hypothetical use of large doses of vitamins fits with our current understanding of the importance of oxidation by free radicals in our tissues. Studies of atherosclerosis in animal models have, in some cases, shown that antioxidant supplements can inhibit the progression of the disease. The risk of taking high doses of these vitamins was thought to be very low, so presumably there was no downside. So well-believed was this theory, in fact, that at a symposium at the American College of Cardiology's annual meeting eight years ago, the session chair, a well-known cardiovascular epidemiologist from Yale, asked the cardiologists attending the session how many of them took high doses of certain vitamins every day—more the half the audience raised their hands!

The vitamins used in the hope of preventing or treating heart disease include C, E, B6, B12, folic acid, and beta-carotene, and are discussed below, along with a look at the role of niacin in treating certain symptoms.

Vitamin C (ascorbic acid)

Vitamin C inhibits the oxidation by free radicals that leads to inflammation and atherosclerosis. In the large National Health and Nutrition Survey in the United States, eating a diet rich in vitamin C was associated with a reduced risk of heart attack. When this finding is considered with the finding of low vitamin C levels in patients with heart disease compared to healthy people, one might suppose that vitamin C would be heart protective. The problem, of course, is that dietary sources of vitamin C, including fresh fruits and vegetables, contain a host of other chemicals that might be cardioprotective, and there are no clinical trials to date that look at vitamin C supplements and heart attack risk. The usual dose used by "believers" is 500 to 1,000mg a day as compared to the RDA of 75 to 90mg a day. There is no evidence from clinical trials that indicates that vitamin C is effective, and doses often get close to the 2,000mg a day, above which there is a safety concern.

Recommendation: My suggestion here is to eat a diet rich in vitamin C, such as a Mediterranean diet, and not to use high-dose supplements.

Vitamin E (alpha-tocopherol)

Vitamin E is an antioxidant that is actually part of the LDL cholesterol particle, and may impart to that particle a resistance to oxidation. Case-cohort and observations studies, such as the Nurses Health Study conducted by the epidemiologists at Harvard Medical School, noted that higher consumption of vitamin E was associated with a reduced risk of heart disease, and one trial, done in England, noted a reduction in nonfatal heart attacks, but not in overall cardiac death, in patients supplemented with vitamin E.

Two large clinical trials have, in effect, put an end to the vitamin E supplement for heart disease. In one, called the HOPE trial, more then 8,500 men and women without heart disease received either a drug (an ACE inhibitor called Ramipril), 400 IU (International Units) of vitamin E, or a placebo over a four-to-six-year period. Vitamin E was no better than the placebo with regard to heart events. The second study referred to was the GISSI study of over 10,000 patients with heart disease. This study showed no benefit of 300 IU of vitamin E a day. The other arm of this trial, as discussed in the chapter on diet, was a 1g fish oil capsule a day, which did reduce mortality and sudden death. Of most importance is a recent study of patients with heart disease given vitamin E at 800 IU, which was stopped because of a *higher* heart attack rate in the vitamin E group as compared to the placebo.

Recommendation: Although there may be more scientific information forthcoming, for the moment no one should take more than 400 IU of vitamin E a day. In fact, there is no reason with regard to heart disease to take vitamin E at all, although there is hope, not confirmed in clinical trials, that it does have a positive effect on a specific form of eye disease (macular degeneration) and Alzheimer's disease.

Beta-carotene

Beta-carotene is a powerful antioxidant and was chosen at the start of the Physicians Health Study to be the substance studied alongside aspirin (one beta-carotene tablet every other day versus one aspirin every other day versus a placebo). Aspirin worked, beta-carotene did not. Additionally, subsequent studies were halted when it became apparent that beta-carotene supplementation increased lung cancer rates and, in one study, heart attack rates.

Recommendation: Beta-carotene supplements should not be used.

Folic Acid, B6, and B12

Folic acid accompanied by B6 and B12 act as cofactors to the enzymes that reduce homocysteine levels in our blood. Elevated homocysteine levels have been linked to up to a fourfold increase in heart attacks in population studies, and increased intake of folic acid has been linked to a reduced incidence of heart disease. Additionally, folic acid may have a direct positive impact on endothelial function. In one clinical trial, folic acid plus B12 and B6 supplementation was shown to lower the rate of closure of coronary stents after angioplasty. There are no completed clinical trials of these supplements in primary and secondary prevention heart attacks, but they are used by most cardiologists for patients with elevated homocysteine levels. Folic acid supplements are used in the range of 800 to 2000mg. There is no evidence that justifies self-treatment with these vitamins.

The recently completed Norwegian Vitamin Trial (NOVIT), presented at the European Society of Cardiology Congress in 2005, looked at the effect of treating heart attack patients with folic acid, B6, or both. It has changed the thinking with regard to folic acid supplements for elevated homocysteine. Folic acid lowered homocysteine but did not reduce second heart attacks or strokes, and when folic acid and B6 were taken together, the second heart attack rate *increased* by 20 percent.

Recommendation: Discuss taking folic acid (alone) with your doctor, but do not take folic acid and B6 together.

Niacin

Niacin in doses of 1,000 to 3,000mg a day is a "medication" (since as noted elsewhere, these amounts are 20 to 60 times more than the amount of niacin contained in most multivitamin pills) that will reduce LDL cholesterol, raise HDL cholesterol, and lower triglycerides. Taken alone, and in combination with a statin, there is good evidence from clinical trials that niacin decreases the incidence of heart attacks and the rates of cardiac death. Common side effects include flushing, itching, and stomach acid symptoms. The flushing can be prevented or reduced by taking an aspirin one hour before the niacin or by using a prescription niacin preparation that is released slowly into the intestines. Niacin, especially in high doses and in a slow-release form, can result in some toxicity to the liver that is reversed when niacin is stopped. The recent introduction of an extended-release form of niacin, which is taken at night, has in a number of my patients been effective at improving lipids and has not been associated with liver abnormalities. Beware, however, of buying "no-flush niacin" over the counter. It is frequently a slightly different chemical (inositol), which produces very little real niacin in your body and has no effect on your lipids!

Recommendation: Niacin should be considered a drug to be prescribed by your physician to treat abnormal lipids, and it should be monitored with appropriate blood tests. There is no data that supports taking high doses as a supplement to prevent heart disease without a physician's input and the blood tests to check for its effect on your lipids and to detect any liver problems.

ALTERNATIVE TREATMENTS FOR HEART DISEASE

As noted earlier in the chapter and in previous chapters, certain alternative treatments, including various forms of meditation and prayer, are highly beneficial in a New Rules program to outlive heart disease. One popular treatment—chelation therapy— is not beneficial and should be avoided. Details follow.

Meditation

Using mediation in a program to prevent and treat heart disease is now mainstream medicine, especially when it is combined with yoga and the slow rhythmic exercise tai chi. Medication and yoga are a part of the Diet Heart Program developed and studied by Dr. Dean Ornish. In the United States meditation is most commonly taught and practiced as either Transcendental Mediation (TM), Mindfulness Meditation, or the Relaxation Response.

Transcendental Mediation involves the focus on one object, such as the sensation of breathing or a sound or phrase that is repeated, termed a mantra. A passive attitude is maintained throughout the process. If distracting thoughts arise, they are to be disregarded, and attention refocused on the breathing or the manta. TM is taught and practiced in 20-minute periods performed twice daily. TM involves no change in lifestyle or personal beliefs or any specific physical activities.

Mindfulness Meditation, also referred to as vipassana or as insight meditation, involves the pointed attention to breathing or mantra, but instead of ignoring outside thoughts or ideas, it invites the meditator to observe and examine them in a passive, nonjudgmental manner with a "distance" between the meditator and his or her thoughts, feelings, and observations. It is thought that the observations of one's thoughts in this mindful and accepting manner allow the individual to approach a stressful situation without the automatic engagement of negative thinking.

The Relaxation Response, developed from observations of Eastern meditation techniques and studied by Dr. Herbert Benson, utilizes the focus on breathing and a mantra (usually a simple number that is repeated slowly in our minds) as well as a visual mantra, a simple object seen in our mind against a blank or monochromatic background. The method is easily taught (Dr. Benson's book on the subject is sufficient to master this technique) and can be performed for very short periods several times during the day, especially when one is feeling stressed.

Clinical studies and some clinical trials, usually involving TM, have demonstrated reduction in blood pressure in hypertensive men and women, a reduction in the blood levels of stress hormones such as cortisol, and the down regulation of the sympathetic nervous system—our fight-or-flight response system. One intriguing study actually documented a reduction in ischemia, the oxygen shortage to the heart that causes pain, during exercise in patients with heart disease and angina pectoris who had engaged in regular meditation. Studies of groups assigned to meditation versus a placebo activity have noted an overall improvement in psychosocial well being. Some studies have noted, however, that mediation can invoke negative emotions and reactions in some subjects.

Recommendation: Meditation is clearly beneficial for most of us, impacting such factors as stress and anxiety, which can have negative cardiac consequences, and improving our sense of psychosocial well being. The only adverse events are negative feelings while meditating or afterward. As with most things, it is not good for everyone. If it doesn't feel right—if the practice seems to increase stress and anxiety instead of reduce it—then don't do it.

Prayer

Prayer is not, in fact, an alternative therapy for most of us; it is part of our daily lives. A survey published in the *Journal of the American Medical Association* that was conducted in 1996 revealed that 96 percent of Americans believe in God, 90 percent pray, and 40 percent had attended a religious service in the week prior to the survey interview. People who do not believe in a higher being and in prayer are in the minority. Prayer can, of course, take many forms and have many purposes, but for consideration of its effect on cardiovascular disease, we focus on "healing prayer" that asks for a good outcome in a specific medical situation. This kind of prayer is called intercessory prayer (we are asking God to intercede). When the prayer is for someone not present at the time of the prayer, we use the term remote- or distant intercessory prayer.

There have been three carefully designed studies of distant intercessory prayer for patients admitted to the hospital with heart disease, and the results are fascinating! The first study was conducted about 15 years ago at San Francisco General Hospital's coronary care unit. Almost 400 patients consented to a study in which they would either be assigned to be prayed for by born-again Christians, or to a control group, for whom no prayers would be said. Those saying the prayers were given only the patients' first names, diagnoses, and clinical updates. The patients, doctors, and other medical staff were not told who was in the prayer group. Using a clinical scoring system to see how well they did during their stay, and comparing the number of serious complications that occurred, the group being prayed for was found, at the end of the study, to have had a 15 to 25 percent better outcome in the hospital, which was determined to be statistically significant.

A second, larger study of more than 1,000 patients was performed at the Mid-America Heart Institute and published in 1999. In this study the CCU patients, doctors, and medical staff were not even told of the study and the intercessors were only given the first name of a patient and told to pray for a speedy recovery without complications. The prayed-for group again did significantly better, with a 10 percent better clinical score and 10 percent fewer serious complications.

The third study was conducted in the CCU at the Mayo Clinic and enrolled 400 patients in the prayer and no-prayer groups. In this study there was no significant difference in the hospital course of the two groups.

Although the impact of intercessory prayer remains uncertain and is the subject of ongoing studies, there is very little doubt about the value of prayer for the patient. Several studies have consistently shown that people who participate in religious services and believe in God have fewer heart attacks (perhaps in part because of the enhanced social support implicit in an organized religious group with group prayer), and that patients undergoing cardiac surgery who believe and pray have better outcomes.

Recommendation: For most of us, then, who believe in God and/or subscribe to a religion, praying is a healthy practice with regard to heart health, and our prayers and the knowledge that our loved ones are praying for us will help us through heart surgery and other procedures.

Homeopathy

This is a unique form of medical treatment that makes no sense in terms of Western science, but has become more popular in the

United States over the past decade, and is in widespread use in India and some European countries. It was developed in the eighteenth century by Samuel Hahnemann. He observed that a high dose of certain medications produced symptoms similar to specific diseases, and that lower doses of these same medications were effective in treating the symptoms of the disease. His first observation was of the drug quinine, which in high doses produced fever and chills similar to malaria, but in lower doses was effective in treating the disease. He called this relationship the principle of similars. His second observation was that the more the dilution and shaking, the more powerful was its clinical effect, which he named the principle of dilutions. The homeopathic preparations thought to be most potent were so dilute that they were unlikely to contain even a single molecule of the original substance, which doesn't make scientific sense. There are, however, a number of clinical trials that suggest a clinical effect of certain preparations for patients with colds, earaches, and digestive complaints. The homeopathic preparations may be prescribed by a homeopathic doctor or may be purchased in health food stores.

Recommendation: In general, homeopathic preparations are used to improve mood, energy, sleep, and overall well-being for heart patients. These highly diluted solutions pose no risk of dangerous interactions with standard medications. The only risk of homeopathy is that the patient may not bring his symptoms to the attention of his physician.

Chelation Therapy

Almost half a million people a year, at an annual estimated cost exceeding $400 million, undergo chelation therapy two or three times a week for periods of one to three months. The process involves the infusion, via a catheter placed in an arm vein, of a solution that contains the substance EDTA, vitamin C, selected B vitamins, and magnesium. EDTA, an accepted treatment for lead poisoning, will bind to heavy metals in our blood, including calcium, and cause them to be excreted in our urine. The concept, when this treatment was first introduced, was that removing calcium from the blood would shrink atherosclerotic plaques that were thought to need calcium to develop. The link between plaque and blood calcium levels has been clearly disproved and such major heart organizations as the American Heart Association and the American College of Cardiology strongly warn people not to undergo this treatment. There are, however, a few small clinical trials that have suggested that patients with atherosclerotic disease of the leg arteries showed improvement in their walking time after undergoing chelation therapy. On the basis of these studies, the National Institutes of Health (NIH) has initiated a clinical trial of chelation therapy.

Recommendation: Do not undergo this treatment. I am concerned that repeated intravenous punctures and infusions are opportunities for serious infection. I will revisit this recommendation after the NIH publishes the results of its trial.

THE NEW RULES–APPROVED USE OF COMPLEMENTARY MEDICINES AND ALTERNATIVE TREATMENTS: A SUMMARY

1. Alternative therapies that are continually presented in the media and by friends and family need to be considered carefully before use as treatments or for prevention of heart disease.
2. With the exception of the vitamin niacin as prescribed by a doctor for low HDL and high triglycerides, high doses of antioxidant vitamins and other supplements are not, according to today's best science, effective in

our New Rules program to outlive heart disease. In some instances, for example, with vitamin E and beta-carotene, they may actually increase cardiac risk.

3. Including garlic cloves in our diets, if we enjoy the taste, may be beneficial and is a reasonable strategy.

4. Red yeast rice is essentially the statin lovastatin (Mevacor), but it is not prepared in a controlled setting and runs the risk of its being adulterated with a toxic substance and thus providing an indeterminate dose of the statin. It makes no sense to take this product when a regulated, carefully prepared dose-specific form of the drug is available.

5. No one, at present, should undergo chelation therapy for heart disease.

6. Homeopathic preparations pose no risk, but failing to discuss the symptoms you're treating with your physician does! Be sure to mention those symptoms—and your nontraditional treatment of them—to your doctor if you want to ensure your heart's health.

7. All of us should consider mediation if we find it a positive experience. For those of us who believe in God and pray, we should not be surprised to learn that prayer has been shown to be a heart-healthy strategy for outliving heart disease.

KEEP UP WITH THE LATEST THERAPIES IN TREATING HEART DISEASE

Even with the best program and lifestyle to prevent heart disease, many of us will still develop atherosclerosis as we age. Knowing about the most advanced tests and undergoing certain procedures *at the right time* will allow us to live longer and healthier lives. Testing, when appropriate, is a critical part of the program to outlive heart disease.

This New Rules chapter presents the "need-to-know" information about important tests and procedures your doctor may—or should—perform, and the rationale your doctor will use in recommending one set of tests over another. This chapter is a bit more detailed than the others, but you need this information to outlive heart disease, especially if you already have heart disease.

The chapter begins with the tests that should be ordered or performed in your doctor's office as part of your initial cardiac evaluation, and then addresses the noninvasive tests that can detect significant coronary artery disease and more precisely determine your risk of a heart attack. Next, the chapter discusses what's involved in coronary angiography, the invasive test that is still the "gold standard" to determine the extent and location of the major atherosclerotic plaques in our coronary arteries. It is a necessary procedure when it is the medically right time to determine if coronary bypass surgery or angioplasty with stenting is called for. Also, newer tests, including Computerized Tomographic (CT) angiography and Magnetic Resonance Imaging (MRI) angiography, are now available in certain hospital centers and even some cardiology offices. These will replace invasive coronary artery angiograms for many of us, though not all of us, because of these tests' limitations, which I will outline below. CT and MRI angiography are still new and cardiologists are still learning how to use them. I will explain what this means to you in terms of limitations of these tests. Your doctor should clearly lead this process, but knowing the basis of his or her thinking and having a sense of the doctor's treatment choices will make you an educated patient who understands why the procedure is necessary and when it may be necessary to seek a second opinion.

The chapter concludes with additional information about cardiac conditions, including valve dysfunction, arrhythmias, and disease of the heart muscle, and the increasingly common treatments that make it possible for you to outlive your heart disease.

THE INITIAL TESTS AND BASIC FOLLOW-UP TESTS

Many of these first-line tests for assessing your risk of heart attack will be ordered or performed by your doctor. Not all of these initial tests make sense for everyone. The goal is to make you well-enough informed to ask whether a particular test is necessary and to understand your doctor's reasoning in his or her answer.

The Physical Examination

In addition to your blood pressure, pulse, and the usual physical examination, the visit should include two measurements:

- Your height and weight, for the calculation of your BMI
- Your waist, to detect and assess obesity and the body structure that could indicate metabolic syndrome (see New Rule No. 2, beginning on page 26)

Blood Tests

Blood should be drawn only if you have fasted from dinner the night before, so that the analysis can be as accurate as possible. Along with the usual complete blood count, examination of your urine, and basic blood profile that addresses kidney and liver function, blood sugar, albumin (a blood protein), and the electrolytes such as sodium, potassium, and calcium, you should have a lipid profile done. This measures total cholesterol, HDL cholesterol, and triglyceride levels, and calculates your LDL cholesterol.

If the fasting blood sugar is over 120 or there is sugar detected in your urine, these tests should be followed by a blood test for Hemoglobin A1C, which reflects the average value of your blood sugar over the past month, and a glucose tolerance test, which requires a blood test every hour for four hours after you drink a special beverage with a high sugar content.

If your cholesterol is high, the follow-up blood studies should also include a test of thyroid function called TSH, or thyroid stimulating hormone. Having an underactive thyroid gland, called hypothyroidism, will sometimes be associated with high cholesterol values, and treatment of the thyroid disorder may result in these values returning to normal.

Electrocardiogram (EKG)

While there is no guideline to indicate when an electrocardio-gram should first be performed and how often it should be fol-lowed up, my practice is to perform one on all patients over the age of 35, and on anyone, regardless of age, who has symptoms of chest pain, shortness of breath, palpitations, dizziness, or feeling faint. Also, patients who describe symptoms that might indicate atypical angina pectoris, such as episodes of extreme tiredness, sweating, or burning or sharp pain in the chest or stomach regions, or an onset of ankle or leg swelling, should have an EKG.

If your risk of developing heart disease has been assessed as being in the intermediate or high-risk group, good cardiac medical practice suggests a repeat of the EKG at least once a year, or more often if new or changing symptoms appear that might reflect a progression of heart disease.

Holter Monitor

When a patient of mine has noted palpitations—either fast, irregular, or unusually strong heartbeats—I will often hook that person up to a device known as a Holter Monitor, which records an EKG continuously for 24 to 48 hours, then plays back its readings in ultrafast mode through a computer that allows me to see what's going on. If there are extra heartbeats, periods of irregular heartbeats, periods of rapid heartbeats called SVT (supraventricular tachycardia), or ventricular tachycardia (abnormal beats that arise in the lower half of the heart, and are of greater concern), then I know whether this patient requires further monitoring and treatment. The Holter Monitor is the size of a small portable radio and is worn on a shoulder strap or clipped to a belt with five wires attached to small adhesive electrodes attached to the chest. Most people do not find it annoying or uncomfortable to wear during the test period.

ADDITIONAL BLOOD TESTS

There are additional tests that I request the lab to perform on blood from my patients who, on coronary heart disease (CHD) risk assessment, score at the intermediate level. Here my goal is to further define their risk and to determine if noninvasive testing is indicated.

C-reactive Protein (CRP)

CRP is a substance in the blood that increases when inflammation is present in the body, and most importantly, the inflammation seen with atherosclerosis and plaque progression. Elevated CRP levels predict heart attacks in much the same way that elevated LDL cholesterol levels do. Studies indicate that the ability of statins to reduce inflammation and lower CRP may be as important in some instances as their ability to lower LDL cholesterol. If my patient's CRP level is elevated and he or she is in an intermediate risk group for developing heart disease, I would, in many instances, start the patient on a statin drug.

Homocysteine

This is an amino acid, one of a group of substances that act for the most part as the building blocks of proteins, and is made in the body by breaking down another amino acid called methionine. Homocysteine is usually converted into other substances immediately, so that the level of homocysteine in our blood is kept low. High levels are toxic to our endothelium and have been found to be predictive of heart attacks. As with LDL cholesterol, the higher the homocysteine level, the greater the risk. Elevated homocysteine can be reduced by taking folic acid with B6 and B12 vitamins, and, until very recently, this was standard therapy. However, the recently completed NOVIT trial, presented at the European Society of Cardiology Congress in 2005, looked at the effect of treating heart attack patients with folic acid, B6, or both. This study has changed the thinking with regard to folic acid supplements for elevated homocysteine. Folic acid lowered homocysteine but did not reduce second heart attacks or strokes, and when folic acid and B6 were taken together, the second heart attack rate increased by 20 percent. Discuss taking folic acid (alone) with your doctor if you have high homocysteine, but do not take folic acid and B6 together.

Lp(a)

Pronounced "L P little a," this substance is a lipoprotein in the same family as LDL cholesterol. This lipoprotein has two distinct halves, one that looks very much like an LDL cholesterol particle and one that is similar to a substance in our blood called plasmin, which the body uses to dissolve clots. We think that Lp(a) can act enough like LDL cholesterol to promote atherosclerosis and that it seems enough like plasmin to the cells of our body to block the effect of our own plasmin and thus promote clot formation in the blood. Elevated levels of Lp(a)—over 30 units—are usually inherited and have been shown to increase risk of heart attacks and strokes in some groups of people, especially if LDL cholesterol is also elevated. To date there are no drugs to reduce Lp(a), other than niacin, which has only a modest effect and can cause bothersome redness and flushing of the skin and stomach symptoms. The strategy to address a high Lp(a) level is to reduce all the other risk factors to as low a level as feasible. It is one of the reasons I will treat patients with borderline elevations of LDL cholesterol down to the new (as of 2004), "optional," indicated low levels of below 70mg/dl. Niacin at doses of 1 to 2 grams a day has been shown to reduce Lp(a) but, at the time of this writing, the value of treating Lp(a) with niacin is unknown.

NEXT LEVEL OF TESTING: NONINVASIVE HEART TESTS

One of the most important questions doctors will ask themselves during clinical evaluation of patients is, "Should I order or perform additional noninvasive (or invasive) tests to detect coronary artery disease, and if so, which one(s)?" Their decisions, of course, are of key importance to you.

What follows is the information I think necessary for patients to have in order to understand what each test actually looks for and what the strengths and the limitations of each test are. This key issue of whether to have the test and what the results might mean is one that, armed with this information, you should discuss directly with your doctor (see New Rule No. 10: Partner with Your Doctor to Reach Your Heart-Health Goals, beginning on page 230).

Unless your symptoms and initial tests indicate significant progression of heart disease, your doctor will probably begin with noninvasive tests for a more complete understanding of your cardiac condition. While he or she could begin with the "gold standard"—angiography—to look for plaques in the heart's arteries, there are some significant risks associated with angiography, and therefore your doctor will most likely order one of the noninvasive tests that might provide the information needed for appropriate treatment while exposing you to less risk.

Noninvasive cardiac tests fit into four groups:

1. Those that *detect a shortage of blood* delivered to the heart by narrowed coronary arteries when exercise or drug-induced "stress" increases the heart's demand for blood;

2. Those that *detect calcium* in the walls of the coronary arteries, which indicates, in almost all instances, the presence and extent of coronary atherosclerosis;

3. Those that *assess the extent of atherosclerosis* in the arterial system of the body, that is, the overall "atherosclerosis burden," not the extent of the process in the coronary arteries;

4. Those that *provide angiogram-like images* of the arteries and of the lumen (the inside opening of the coronary arteries) without the insertion of catheters into the arteries.

Some of the noninvasive tests to find coronary heart disease and, if present, to determine how severe it is, are less accurate in women than in men. Having the right test and having the results interpreted correctly is a crucial issue for women.

Group 1: Tests That Detect a Reduced Blood Flow to a Region of the Heart Muscle During Stress

Exercise EKG Testing

The oldest of the noninvasive tests used to detect atherosclerotic narrowing of the heart arteries, a patient's EKG is measured during increasing levels of treadmill or bicycle exercise until the patient is near exhaustion, has chest pain, or has a change in his or her EKG reading. The most important EKG change is called ST segment depression, which indicates that part of the heart is becoming short of blood and oxygen, usually because of a narrowed coronary artery. There are other reasons that ST segment depression can occur with exercise, such as the patient's taking certain drugs (such as digitalis). On occasion we will see ST segment depression in a patient with normal coronary arteries on angiogram.

These results are called false positives and are more common in people who before the test have only a very small chance of having coronary artery disease (see my description of Bayes Theorum at the end of this chapter to understand why), and in people who are able to do a lot of exercise on the treadmill. Also, false positives are more common in women, partly because many women being tested have a lower likelihood of having heart disease than men of a similar age, and partly because of reasons we don't yet understand. In general, because of false positives, exercise EKG testing is done less often on women. Many doctors do exercise testing with nuclear- or echo-imaging as the first-line test in women.

Exercise Stress Nuclear Imaging

This is an exercise EKG test as described above that also involves an injection of a nuclear isotope at peak exercise and at rest. (The isotope used originally was thallium and so the test is often referred to as a thallium stress test.) This kind of testing can also be performed by substituting an intravenous drug such as Persantine or Adenosine for the exercise. The isotope injection exposes the patient to only a very small amount of radiation, which is almost never an issue (except in women who are or may be pregnant). An area of the heart muscle supplied by a significantly narrowed coronary artery will pick up less isotope during exercise, and thus emit fewer gamma rays in images of the heart that are produced. The location and size of an area of heart muscle that gets relatively less blood during exercise or stress, called a cold spot, is easily noted using software called SPECT, which produces pictures of two-dimensional slices through the heart. These images allow doctors to determine the coronary artery involved, and in some instances, approximately where along the course of that artery the most significant obstruction is. A word of advice with regard to stress nuclear studies: if you plan to fly within two days of the test, ask your doctor for a note stating that you underwent this procedure, as the radiation detectors at airports are now sensitive enough to sound an alarm as you pass through them. So to make your life easier, have the note in your hand.

Exercise Stress Echocardiography

Echocardiography uses high-frequency sound waves to produce echos, or sound waves bounced back from the different parts of the heart, in much in the same ways that ships at sea use sonar to map the ocean floor. The result is pictures of the moving heart, including the chamber walls and the valves between the chambers. Echocardiography also shows the direction and speed of blood flow within the heart. As with exercise EKG testing and exercise nuclear studies, exercise in exercise echocardiography is used to increase the work of the heart and its demand for blood. Areas of the heart wall supplied by narrowed arteries will become ischemic during exercise (or drug-induced stress), and will not contract as well as neighboring areas of heart wall supplied by normal arteries. Comparing the motion of the walls of the heart at rest and at peak exercise will show areas that become ischemic with exercise and indicate which of the heart's arteries are narrowed by coronary heart disease.

It is important to note that the value of this test, usually considered to be equal to a nuclear stress test, is very much based on the training and skill of the cardiologist performing and interpreting the studies. The quality of stress echo studies varies to a greater extent than nuclear studies, and, if this test is the one prescribed for you, you and your physician must be confident in the training and skill of the cardiologist and the laboratory performing it.

Group 2: A Test That Detects Calcium in the Wall of the Coronary Arteries

Electron Beam Computerized Tomographic (often referred to as EBCT) Imaging of Coronary Artery Calcium and a similar calcium detection technique performed with a helical CT X-ray machine

We don't normally have calcium in the walls of our coronary arteries, except in the presence of atherosclerotic plaques. Calcium develops as plaques grow and is more often seen in larger plaques. Imaging calcium with X-ray technology had been a problem, since the heart is continually moving during contraction and relaxation. Precise measurement and localizations have required the technology to get the images in such a short period of time that it effectively "freezes" the heart to get an accurate picture. The advent of ultrafast imaging using the EBCT or the helical CT technology has overcome this barrier and allowed the detection and measurement of the size of calcium deposits in the wall of the coronary arteries. These deposits are scored by a computerized system linked to the camera. The absence of calcium is highly predictive of the absence of coronary obstructions on an angiogram, and of a very low risk of cardiac events. Very high scores predict significant coronary artery disease on coronary angiography. Scores in the intermediate range (the most common outcome in my experience) are frequently followed up with an exercise-, nuclear-, or echocardiography study. The data increasingly support the use of this technique, especially in regard to the more precise calculation of risk, and the decision regarding further testing, for patients in the intermediate range (6 to 20 percent predicted chance of a heart attack death within 10 years). Because this test is not covered by many health insurance carriers, it is not being widely used.

Group 3: A Test That Directly Measures the Extent of Atherosclerosis in the Major Artery That Supplies Blood to the Brain

Carotid Intimal Medial Thickness Measurement by Ultrasound
The process of atherosclerosis takes place between the most inside intimal layer of endothelial cells and the adjacent medial layer of smooth muscle cells in the wall of the artery. (See New Rule No. 2, page 26, for a diagram of the location of atherosclerosis in our blood vessels.) Measuring the thickness of this zone in the wall of the artery by ultrasound is a measurement of the degree of atherosclerosis. Since atherosclerosis is a diffuse process and this measurement is in the carotid artery of the neck (which is close to the skin and thus easily measured with a high degree of accuracy), this test reflects the overall extent of plaque development in an individual. This test does not measure specific plaques, but in most instances the greater the carotid-medial thickness, the more likely the patient is to have many and large plaques in the coronary arteries.

Clinical research over the past several years has supported the use of the carotid artery for assessment of the extent of a patient's atherosclerosis. At present, though, this test is used primarily as a research tool to measure the extent of a patient's overall atherosclerosis and to follow the progression or regression of the disease with treatments that are being researched. The test is not currently paid for by most insurance companies and managed health plans, but I expect it will be widely used and paid for by medical insurance companies in the near future.

Group 4: Tests That Produce Visual Images of the Coronary Arteries

MRI Coronary Angiography and CT Coronary Angiography
Using high resolution X-ray and MRI-generated images of the heart with a fast-enough imaging rate to overcome blurring from the moving heart, doctors are now able to generate pictures of the coronary arteries of the heart that actually look like the arteries! These images are of high-enough quality to detect and measure obstruction caused by atherosclerotic plaques. They are, in fact, amazing images to the current generation of cardiologists. What are now necessary are large clinical trials of patients who have had these studies and subsequent coronary angiograms, so that the correlation of the findings on the noninvasive angiograms can be validated. This information is becoming available very quickly and more studies are confirming that they are clinically reliable. MRI and CT angiography are decreasing the need for invasive coronary angiography, thus rewriting, again, the rules for disease detection! Some centers and even doctors' offices are doing these studies and providing data. The quality of the picture received, though, is highly dependent on the use of new-generation CT units. In addition, the experience and training of the physician reading the study is a critical issue. If you are going to have this study done, ask about both of these issues.

LOOKING AHEAD

Coming in the near future are noninvasive tests that measure the health of the endothelial cells that line our arteries.

Our current understanding of the endothelial cell as the "controller" of the process of atherosclerosis and the vulnerability of our plaques to rupture is the basis of studies that test endothelial function and correlate the findings with future cardiac events. Two observations have made such testing possible. One is the finding that atherosclerosis in the coronary arteries is associated with abnormal endothelial function throughout our blood vessels. We can thus make a general statement about endothelial function in the arteries of the heart by using noninvasive methods in the artery in the arm, which is easily imaged at elbow level and involves less risk than undergoing coronary angiography to directly study the coronary arteries.

The second important finding is the increase in production of nitric oxide by healthy endothelial cells when blood flow is suddenly increased, causing the artery to expand. We produce this effect by blowing up a blood pressure cuff to occlude the artery in the arm for five minutes (which causes the small blood vessels in the arm muscles to dilate), and then releasing the cuff and measuring the resultant increase of blood flow and dilatation of the artery. In the patient without atherosclerosis, the artery will dilate 5 percent more than the measurement obtained at baseline. Less dilation indicates dysfunctional endothelium, which in many clinical settings indicates the active process of atherosclerosis. This study takes 15 to 30 minutes and uses only a blood pressure cuff and an ultrasound probe positioned against the skin on the inside surface of the arm. Abnormal findings are being correlated with later coronary events to measure the extent of atherosclerosis and the vulnerable status of the plaques. At present, measuring the arteries' diameters in a consistent manner is a difficult technique to master and has been limited to research settings.

THE INVASIVE TEST: ANGIOGRAPHY, OR THE "GOLD STANDARD"

Under certain circumstances, your cardiologist will want a more complete understanding of the extent or progression of your coronary artery atherosclerosis and will recommend a coronary angiogram. If we had a perfectly accurate and risk-free test, deciding which test to perform would not be an issue. Unfortunately, we do not. For years, the "gold-standard" test to measure degree of heart disease has been coronary angiography, which provides a high-quality X-ray picture of the inside of the coronary arteries. A hollow catheter, thinner than a drinking straw, is placed, via a needle puncture, into the femoral artery (the large artery at the top of our legs), and then advanced up through the main artery of the body, the aorta, until it reaches the opening of the two main coronary arteries. Here, a clear solution containing iodine that shows up on X-ray (called a dye, although it is not) is injected into these arteries to produce a high-quality picture of the lumen, the inside opening of the coronary arteries. The downside of this test is the small but real risk of damage to the artery, or a stroke caused by dislodging pieces of plaque with the tip of the catheter, and a rare, but also real, risk of a catastrophic cardiovascular event and death. The benefit of the information gathered is the ability to guide life-prolonging treatment strategies. The benefit of angiography greatly outweighs the real risks of the procedure if there is a reasonable likelihood that coronary artery disease requiring angioplasty or surgery will be found. If coronary angiography were used as a routine screening test on a population of very low-risk patients—those without symptoms, EKG changes, or, in some instances, risk-associated conditions—we would find very little disease and yet expose those patients to most of the risks noted. This would not be good medical practice!

Angiography, therefore, should be performed only when there is a clear likelihood of significant coronary artery disease, or when the symptoms of angina pectoris are increasing, coming on at rest, or associated with important changes on the patient's electrocardiogram. These symptoms describe a potentially dangerous condition referred to as unstable coronary syndrome and provide a good reason to do an immediate coronary angiogram.

FALSE SENSE OF SECURITY

In addition to the risk of the procedure, there is another concern with angiography: a false sense of security that an angiogram provides when it shows only minimal narrowing of the coronary artery. In the early stages of a plaque's growth, the outer wall of the artery at the site of the plaque bulges out to accommodate the mass of the plaque, so the lumen is protected. Thus an angiogram would appear nearly normal despite the existence of a moderate-sized plaque. Also, we've learned that small plaques can frequently be the unstable ones that tend to rupture; the absence of a large obstructing plaque does not necessarily mean that we aren't at risk of a heart attack. An angiographic technique, called intravascular ultrasound, which uses a tiny ultrasound crystal at the tip of a wire threaded through the coronary arteries, is available in many angioplasty laboratories and provides images of specific slices though the artery, showing the size of the plaque and the extent to which it is inside the wall. This test gives us more information than the angiogram, which can only show us how narrow the blood vessel has become. This test, however, involves the same risks as the angiogram and the additional risks associated with threading a wire through the coronary artery. It is thus not routinely used to detect the existence of plaques.

INTERPRETING THE RESULTS OF NONINVASIVE TESTS

After you have undergone one or more of the tests, the critical issue is how they will be interpreted and acted upon by your doctor and you. Being an informed patient at this point is critical to "best care" as you and your doctor face the next pivotal question: "What should happen after I get the results of the test?"

The answers, as is the case in much of cardiac medicine, are often not crystal clear, and should be based in large part on your specific clinical picture. Why are the answers not always clear? Although doctors must rely on noninvasive tests, the results are, as we have discussed, not a perfect way to diagnose the presence or amount of major blockage of the coronary arteries, and frequently will not tell us precisely about the overall extent of the atherosclerotic disease, or provide an accurate and precise prediction as to whether you will have a heart attack in the near future. Interpreting test results is the point at which the science of medicine becomes the art of diagnosis, and when you as a patient must work with your doctor to arrive at an appropriate course of treatment to outlive your heart disease.

How good a given test is at correctly detecting or excluding heart disease as compared to coronary angiography (the invasive gold standard) is determined by its sensitivity and its specificity. The sensitivity of a test refers to how often patients with heart disease on angiography will have a positive test. For example, a test that has 90 percent sensitivity, such as the exercise echocardiogram, or stress nuclear study, with up-to-date equipment and software for SPECT analysis, should be positive in nine out of ten patients with coronary artery disease. The specificity of a test refers to how many patients without heart disease will have a negative test—again, 90 percent means that nine out of ten people without coronary artery disease will have a negative test.

On the flip side, however, this test result means that one in ten patients with coronary artery disease will have a negative test and be missed, and one in ten patients without disease will have a positive test and possibly undergo an unwarranted angiogram. This one-in-ten risk is only one of the factors that you and your doctor need to consider when discussing the results of these tests.

The other factor is a statistical principle called Bayes Theorum, named after the Anglican priest in England who described and proved it. Simply put, this theorem mathematically described and determined that the ability of an imperfect test to correctly detect or exclude a finding (in this case, coronary artery disease) is determined in part by the likelihood of coronary disease in the population tested. Noninvasive testing is thus of increasing clinical value, and more likely to accurately detect or exclude disease, in populations in which disease is more prevalent. To put it differently, the more likely you and I are to have heart disease, the more accurate the test will be in detecting or excluding heart disease. Thus, testing healthy asymptomatic 50-year-old women will be of significantly less clinical value than testing 60-year-old men with chest pain during stress. I spend a good deal of time "proving" this theorem to my cardiology fellows, since it doesn't make sense when you first hear about it—but it is indeed true!

These studies have another important role besides detecting or excluding disease, and that is risk assessment, which is to correctly predict a patient's chances of having a cardiac event in a given period of time. Exercise EKG testing can be of real value in this regard. A formula that factors in how long a patient exercises, chest pain felt during exercise, and presence of ST segment depression on the exercise EKG was developed at Duke University and so is named the Duke Treadmill Index. Your Duke Treadmill Index will predict, with reasonable accuracy, your chances of dying of heart disease in the next 10 years. This is of course a group prediction and should be figured in with your other risk factors to arrive at an estimate of your chance or likelihood of a cardiac event or death.

It is exactly that risk of having a cardiac event that is an important factor, possibly the most important factor, in deciding whether to go forward with more invasive testing and therapies. The more accurately your risk is assessed, the better the decisions that can be made with regard to outliving your heart disease. If you have a very low risk and no important symptoms, then *any* test, procedure, or even drug with risk of an adverse event is often a bad idea. If you have intermediate risk, then further testing to determine the need for angioplasty, surgery, and the use of drugs that have been shown to reduce risk are often appropriate and may indeed represent your best chances for outliving heart disease! If your risk is high and you have symptoms of coronary artery disease, angiography may be an appropriate *first* step.

In this context, one role of noninvasive testing becomes clear. In patients with intermediate risk, who represent a population with an intermediate prevalence of disease and symptoms or compelling risk factors, noninvasive testing can select, by virtue of positive testing, those of us at increased risk in whom invasive angiography may be indicated, and in whom aggressive use of medications and lifestyle prevention strategies can be lifesaving.

As outlined in earlier chapters, physicians estimate our CHD 10-year endpoint risk using the Framingham risk calculation scoring system. We accumulate points based on our age and sex, total cholesterol, HDL cholesterol, tobacco-smoking history, and systolic blood pressure. We then use points to assign ourselves to a 10-year risk group. A 10-year risk below 6 percent is considered low risk, and so further testing in apparently healthy individuals, unless indicated by symptoms or significantly atherosclerotic-associated conditions such as diabetes, is not advised. If your risk is 6 to 20 percent, then further refinement of this intermediate risk downward or upward based on noninvasive testing may be advised. If your risk is greater than 20 percent, then, in many instances, noninvasive testing is necessary, even in the absence of symptoms or associated conditions.

The bottom line is this: you should discuss with your doctor noninvasive testing, preferably exercise nuclear testing in an experienced clinical laboratory with a contemporary nuclear camera, if:

- you have symptoms that suggest coronary artery disease;
- you have significant associated conditions and are a man over age 50 or a woman over age 60;
- your Framingham risk score represents a 10-year cardiac-event risk of over 6 percent.

The goals of testing are the detection of coronary artery disease and the more precise assessment of your 10-year event risk (up or down).

Calcium score testing has been shown in studies of intermediate risk populations to provide additional information of patient risk of a cardiac event and may be incorporated into clinical practice as soon as data from larger groups of patients from multiple centers are reported and analyzed. The data as of this writing support a very low risk in patients with low calcium scores and a graded increase in risk with increasing scores. Calcium score testing should be discussed with your physician, and if you choose to have EBCT, then expect to have further testing (stress nuclear or stress echo) if calcium scores are intermediate or high.

For now, noninvasive testing following Framingham risk assessment should be stress testing with nuclear or echocardiography imaging, as appropriate.

WHEN INVASIVE PROCEDURES ARE INDICATED

At some point, many of us will have some form of heart disease that can be significantly improved by successful surgery, angioplasty, or other kinds of invasive procedures. Outliving heart disease is often made possible by having *the right procedure at the right time*. The right time is that point when a successful procedure will improve how well and how long we live at a risk that is significantly less than the risk of doing nothing. Surgery or angioplasty performed before this point doesn't make sense, even in our New Rules context, since the risk is not clearly balanced by the gain. However, waiting too long to have a necessary invasive procedure forces us to accept more risk of the disease progressing, along with the greater risk involved in having the procedure performed at a later time.

This section provides the information you need to work effectively with your physician (usually your cardiologist, if you have arrived at this point) in deciding which procedure to have, when it should be done, and where and by whom it should be done. In addition to coronary artery bypass surgery and angioplasty, I will refer to other important procedures that will play an important part in outliving your heart disease and which are more fully discussed in the last chapter, entitled "Partner with Your Doctor to Reach Your Heart-Health Goals."

Considering Angioplasty and Bypass Surgery

Based on the evidence gathered from large, well-designed studies of coronary artery bypass graft surgery and a smaller number of studies of angioplasty, these two invasive procedures should be considered when *one* of the following conditions is met:

1. You have chest pain on exertion or stress (angina) that has been shown definitely to be due to coronary artery disease, is causing enough pain or reduction of your activity to have a negative impact on the quality of your life, and cannot be eradicated or significantly reduced by medications.

2. You have significant obstruction in all three main coronary arteries.

3. You have significant obstruction in two coronary arteries and evidence of already damaged heart muscle.

4. You have a significant obstruction in the left main coronary artery that can be seen on your coronary angiography. In this one case, obstructions that reduce the lumen of the left main coronary artery by greater than 50 percent are considered significant, compared with the 70 percent that we need to be significant in the three main coronary arteries.

5. You have a damaged heart valve that needs repair or replacement and also have (on your coronary angiography) significant obstruction of a coronary artery.

6. You go to your doctor or to the emergency room with *unstable coronary syndrome*, such as chest pain at rest, associated with changes on your EKG and elevations of the cardiac markers that indicate damage

to heart muscle cells, and your coronary angiography shows a significant coronary lesion.

Although not based on solid clinical evidence yet, and especially with regard to angioplasty, the following are also commonly used indications for surgery or angioplasty.

7. You have significant disease in two coronary artery vessels and medical therapy does not completely eradicate angina during usual activity levels.
8. You have two or fewer coronary arteries with significant lesions that produce ischemia on a stress imaging test and you want to continue to perform very intensive exercise or exercise in difficult environments (for example, high-altitude mountain climbing).

The point I am making here is that there are specific combinations of prior heart disease, symptoms of heart disease, and findings on coronary angiography that describe people who will live better and longer with heart surgery, and in many instances, angioplasty. Having coronary artery disease that does not meet one of the above criteria is not a good reason to have surgery or angioplasty. There is too much risk for too little gain!

CORONARY ARTERY BYPASS GRAFT SURGERY

This major operation is now performed so often in the United States that even doctors tend to forget what a big and complex procedure it is. For the average patient, the risk of dying or having a serious complication, such as a stroke, is less than 1 in 200 cases. The average hospital stay is three to four days. In most cases the patient is able to sit in a chair with most tubes and wires having been removed, by the day after surgery. Innovations in surgical technique, medical management of the heart during surgery, and patient care in the important 12 to 24 hours after surgery have brought CABG risk down to this low level. (Considering the open-heart surgeries I saw in the 1970s, this improvement in risk is still rather remarkable to me.)

The purpose of this surgery is very simple: to create a "bypass" around a very large atherosclerotic plaque that is blocking the coronary artery. The bypass can be made using your own artery, usually the mammary artery that travels in the wall of your chest, or by using a vein taken from your leg (specifically, the saphenous vein). The mammary artery is a good choice for creating a bypass graft, since it is almost always free of atherosclerosis and has a very low likelihood of becoming blocked in the years following surgery. Saphenous veins, in contrast, have a risk of becoming blocked in the years following surgery.

The traditional and in most instances still-standard CABG operation involves putting the patient on a heart-lung machine that enriches the blood with oxygen and pumps it around the body without the heart, so that the surgeon can cut and sew in a nonmoving heart. The past seven years have seen the development, and now the widespread successful use, of "off-pump" CABG, in which the heart is left beating, and the heart-lung machine is not used. The surgeon, using a device to stabilize the area in which he or she is sewing, performs the operation on the beating heart. Clinical studies are showing that off-pump surgery takes less time and results in an equally successful surgery when compared with on-pump surgery *when the surgeon is experienced in this technique*. It is hoped that by avoiding the use of the heart-lung machine, the complications, especially those involving mental function after surgery, will be reduced. So far, this important issue remains undetermined.

Questions to Ask When Considering CABG or Angioplasty

The decision to have bypass surgery, especially now that angioplasty with the coated stents described later in this chapter is widely available, should be based on the following issues, presented here as questions that you and your physician should discuss.

Will I need to have a valve repaired or replaced at the same time as the bypass grafts are performed?
If you have a valve, usually the mitral or aortic valve on the left side of the heart, that will need repair or replacement, then you will need open heart surgery; the CABG can and should be done at the same time.

Will I need to have three or more coronary arteries bypass grafted, one of which is the left anterior descending artery that travels down the front of the heart? Or has my heart already been damaged by a heart attack or other condition so that its ejections fraction (a calculation of how well the heart pumps blood) is well below normal and at least two arteries will require bypass grafts?
Strong clinical evidence shows that CABG surgery in patients with obstructions of three major blood vessels, or in two major blood vessels when the heart muscle has been damaged, result in the patient living significantly longer. This is especially true when the left anterior descending (known as LAD) artery is bypassed with the patient's internal mammary artery.

Is my left main coronary artery obstructed?
When the short left main coronary artery, which splits to become the two major left coronary arteries (the LAD and the circumflex artery), is significantly obstructed, the risk of dying from a heart

attack is very high and CABG to the LAD and circumflex arteries is urgently required. Studies from selected centers have shown that you can have angioplasty and insert a stent at the left main obstruction with reasonably low risk, but CABG is still, at present, the best choice.

Are the obstructing plaques in a place in the coronary artery that would make angioplasty difficult or risky?
This is an important question, since the goal is to address all the major blockages and you don't want to have angioplasty if there is a good chance that one or more of the vessels will not be opened or if the risk of a complication during angioplasty for one of the obstructing plaques is too great. If one of these scenarios is the case, then CABG surgery may well be the better choice.

You need to address with your cardiologist the possibility of having a procedure and the reason for CABG over angioplasty, or visa versa. Remember to ask the "golden question": What about trying maximum medical and lifestyle treatment, including statins to lower cholesterol down into the 70mg/dl range? This question is especially important if you only have one or two arteries blocked, normal heart muscle, and mild to moderate angina that can be controlled with medications.

I cannot say this too often: if medical and lifestyle–change therapy is not an option and if surgery is recommended, then be sure you fit into one of the eight categories noted. If not, then a good long discussion and explanation, and probably a second opinion, are smart ideas. If you are an appropriate patient for CABG surgery, you need to address with your doctor *and the surgeon* the issues of off-pump surgery and the use of mammary artery bypass grafts for the LAD and, if there is not a contraindication, the use of both mammary arteries for all the grafts. It is very important that you choose a surgeon who has extensive experience (hundreds of cases and at least several years' experience) with off-pump CABG cases. Less-experienced surgeons may not successfully bypass difficult vessels in the back of the heart. Also, surgeons differ with regard to their comfort and experience using both the right and left mammary arteries to do all arterial bypasses. Often the best information about a surgeon will come from your cardiologist.

> The benefits of coronary artery bypass surgery and angioplasty are, in some instances, less favorable for women than for men, due, in part, to the greater amount of heart disease and the older age of women undergoing these procedures as compared to men. Decisions about angioplasty and surgery always require careful evaluation and thinking, but even more so in women!

Percutaneous Trans Coronary Angioplasty (often referred to as PTCA, angioplasty, or interventional cardiology) with Stent Deployment
Before stents were developed, balloon angioplasty was done as a stand-alone procedure and involved placing a very small catheter with a built-in balloon into a coronary artery. The balloon was then inflated at the site of the obstruction and pushed the plaque material into the wall of the artery to open the lumen. The patient felt almost instant relief of angina symptoms. While this procedure was successful and had a reasonably low complication rate, the vessel would sometimes reclose immediately, requiring emergency reopening or, in some instances, emergency bypass surgery. Additionally, in about one-third of patients, the vessel would renarrow part or all of the way in the six months following the procedure—a process called restenosis, necessitating repeat PTCA. When small metal stents that could be placed over a balloon (which would be inflated to hold open the vessel) at the

Sirolimus Coated Stent

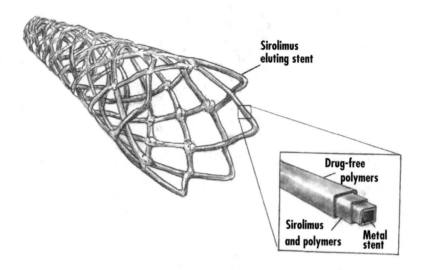

Sirolimus
eluting stent

Drug-free
polymers

Sirolimus
and polymers

Metal
stent

site of the angioplasty were developed, the problem of immediate closure was resolved, but the issue of six-month restenosis due to tissue growth remained. The final improvement that has revolutionized this technique was coating the stents with substances that inhibit local tissue growth.

The use of coated stents has reduced the problem of restenosis from one-third of stent patients to 5 to 10 percent or less. Angioplasty with coated stents is now being used to treat patients who only two to three years ago were recommended for CABG surgery. PTCA with coated stents usually takes about one to two hours and the patient is usually discharged the next day without residual pain. Drug-coated stents have been associated with acute clots at the site of the stent and with heart attacks if the drug clopidigril (Plavix) is not taken for one full year following the stent placement. This can be a problem, since Plavix needs to be stopped for at least five days before any significant surgery to avoid excessive bleeding. The risks and the benefits of a coated stent should be discussed with the cardiologist. In some instances they are clearly the right choice (in patients who are diabetic, for example, or those in whom a stent needs to be placed in a very small section of the coronary artery), and in some instances they may not be (those who anticipate surgery during the next six months to one year). It is important to note, however, that serious complications of the PTCA procedure are still about the same as that of CABG surgery (over 1 in 100 cases).

Despite the ease for the patient and the now very good long-term rates of remaining open, PTCA with stents must meet the criteria of improving symptoms when medications have failed, or of improving the coronary anatomy in situations where CABG has been shown to improve and prolong life. PTCA is, in clinical practice, used by some physicians in situations where there is no evidence that opening a narrowed artery will make the patient feel better or live longer. In some of these situations, future studies may show that this is good medical therapy, but for now we are subjecting the patient (you!) to the risk without evidence of benefit.

Note: It is not uncommon that patients have angioplasty for obstruction of a single vessel that was initially detected by exercise testing or exercise imaging, or suggested by having only stable angina (chest pain brought on repeatedly at the same levels of exertion). There is no evidence that we are doing a good thing in terms of quality or duration of life by having these patients undergo PTCA in this reasonably low-risk situation. When patients see me for second opinions before such a procedure, I counsel them to defer the procedure and do the following instead:

• take appropriate medications such as aspirin;

- aggressively treat their risk factors, including lowering LDL cholesterol to below 70mg/dl;
- engage in a structured cardiac exercise program;
- work with their physician to increase angina medications to resolve or significantly diminish their chest pain.

Beware: This wonderful technique has led well-meaning cardiologists on occasion to open vessels at a small but real risk without good evidence that the procedure is doing any real good. If this procedure is recommended for you, get a second opinion from a cardiologist who is familiar with the latest data about its advantages and risks.

THE OTHER FACES OF HEART DISEASE

Heart disease for most of us, as discussed in this book, refers to coronary heart disease, coronary artery atherosclerosis leading to a heart attack, and sudden death. For an increasing number of us, our heart disease may instead be due to:

- Cardiac arrhythmias
- Heart valves that dysfunction
- Disease of the heart muscle called cardiomyopathy

These conditions, along with coronary heart disease and high blood pressure, are increasingly leading to the most important "other face" of heart disease—heart failure. The strategies that are effective in these instances and that optimize our chances of outliving coronary disease are the same as those that comprise the New Rules. They are:

- Prevention
- Prompt diagnosis with best tests, given in a timely manner
- The best treatment available once the extent of the condition is understood
- Appropriate noninvasive or invasive procedures, where needed

CARDIAC ARRHYTHMIAS

Normally, the electrical impulse that controls the way the heart beats starts in the upper area of the heart, called the sinus node, and travels down the heart in an orderly way. This is called normal sinus rhythm. When this process is altered, the changed pattern of heartbeats is termed arrhythmia.

Arrhythmias can occur in many forms. If the electrical signal is stopped or stalled and the heart rate is slowed, or if long pauses occur between beats, the arrhythmia is called a heart block. In some instances a heart block is treated with a *pacemaker,* a small device (about the size of a stack of three half-dollars) placed under the skin whose wires are inserted through a vein in the right atrium and ventricle. The pacemaker will sense the electrical activity of the atria and the ventricles and will stimulate either chamber to "beat" in the case of a block or a long pause. When extra or early heart beats that do not originate in the sinus node occur, they are named for their heart chamber of origin; for instance, APCs are atrial premature contractions, and VPCs are ventricular premature contractions. Occasional APCs and VPCs occur commonly in all of us and usually do no harm. Recurring extra heartbeats that arise in the atria can result in a fast rhythm that often requires treatment. Of greatest concern is a period of continued extra heartbeats that arise in the lower part of the heart, the ventricles. These extra beats can cause symptoms and in some cases may be a harbinger of ventricular fibrillation (the wavy line we see on the monitors on the emergency medicine TV shows), which, if not interrupted, will lead quickly to death.

The rapid regular beating that usually starts in the atrial chambers at the top of the heart, called SVT, can sometimes be corrected with medications, but are now often set right by a procedure called electrophysiology, which employs radio frequency ablation. In this procedure, wires are placed in the heart in the same manner as in a cardiac catheterization. The "short circuits" in the conduction pathway responsible for the arrhythmia are identified and destroyed with a small energy pulse.

When the impulses are disorganized in the atrium of the heart, they stimulate the ventricles to beat in an irregular fashion, resulting in an arrhythmia called atrial fibrillation. This is the most frequent and important arrhythmia. With atrial fibrillation, the heart rate is often fast and is always irregular. The goal in this case is twofold: to bring the heart rate into a good range, and to lower the high risk of a stroke due to blood clots forming in the left atrium chamber and breaking off to travel in the blood to block a vessel in the brain. (The risk of stroke in a patient with atrial fibrillation can be as high as five times that of someone with normal heart rhythm!) Coumadin, a drug that reduces the clotting process in the blood, is used in appropriate patients to reduce this risk. It is now possible in some patients to use electrophysiology with radio frequency ablation (the same technique that is successful in SVT), to return some patients to normal sinus rhythm. In many regards, this treatment is still new but something you should discuss with your cardiologist periodically, since the growing experience with this treatment has increased its value to selected patients.

When the ventricle is generating its own impulses, instead of receiving the impulses from the atrial chambers at the top of the heart, the result is called ventricular tachycardia, which may cause symptoms such as dizziness or fainting, or may have no symptoms at all. This arrhythmia has a high risk of becoming ventricular fibrillation and leading to sudden death, and is thus often treated with a device called an implantable cardiac defibrillator, which is surgically placed in the same manner as a pacemaker. This device monitors the EKG and, when it detects ventricular tachycardia or ventricular fibrillation, will deliver a shock directly to the heart to terminate this arrhythmia. This small device has proven to dramatically reduce sudden deaths in specific conditions. The evaluation of some heart blocks, of SVT, and of ventricular tachycardia will often involve an electrophysiology study, possibly with one of two treatment methods:

- Radio frequency ablation, which is the use of radio frequency energy at the tip of a catheter to destroy a very small part of the heart muscle, hopefully the abnormal circuit responsible for the SVT, or
- Placement of an automatic cardiac defibrillator

Both methods are performed by an electrophysiologist, that is, a cardiologist with at least one additional year of special training in this technique.

An important New Rules strategy for patients with arrhythmias is to discuss with your doctor whether a referral to an electrophysiologist would be of value.

HEART VALVE DISEASE

Increasingly I am seeing adults, and especially senior patients, who have the symptoms of angina pectoris (chest pain with exercise or emotional stress) or of heart failure (shortness of breath with mild to moderate exercise and swelling of the ankles and legs) in whom the problem is a heart valve that doesn't open fully (stenosis) or close properly (insufficiency/regurgitation). In some cases, these conditions are congenital: the patient was born with valves that were slightly abnormal and worked fine until well into adulthood. In many instances the exact basis for the deterioration of the heart valve is not yet known.

The two most common valve problems are:

1. Calcified stenosis of the aortic valve
2. Degenerative mitral valve insufficiency

In many cases of calcified aortic stenosis, the patient was born with a valve that has only two components instead of the usual three, and over time the abnormal swirling of the blood passing through the valve traumatized the heart valve tissue and resulted in the thickening and calcification of the valve, leading to stenosis. Many patients initially had degenerative mitral valves that easily stretched and bulged backward with each contraction (this is called mitral valve prolapse) and over time, the valve stretched and no longer closed fully, resulting in insufficiency. When the aortic valve doesn't open all the way, the heart has to work harder to pump the blood through a smaller opening. As a result, the heart first thickens, but then becomes weaker, leading to heart failure. With mitral valve insufficiency, much of the blood goes backward into the left atrium with each heartbeat, causing enlargement and weakening of the left ventricle, leading to heart failure and causing atrial fibrillation.

In both valve problems, the heart failure is due to mechanical problems (*not* plaque buildup), and medications are only modestly effective at delaying the onset of heart failure and relieving symptoms. The effective strategy is to fix or replace the heart valve at the right time—that is, before the heart is so damaged that the failure cannot be reversed or the surgery has become too risky. Echocardiography, the technique that uses sonar to produce a picture of the moving heart and the blood within it, is the major test to track the damage to the valve and the heart muscle, and it is often repeated every six months to a year to help in deciding the best time to replace it or, in the case of a mitral valve, possibly to perform surgery to repair it. A cardiac catheterization with coronary angiograms is usually only done at the time that heart valve surgery is being seriously considered.

Heart valve disease can also result in an infection on the heart valve, which will further damage it and cause more insufficiency. This condition is called bacterial endocarditis and is treated with intravenous antibiotics. Rapid diagnosis and treatment will minimize the damage to the heart. The best tests for bacterial endocarditis are echocardiography, which is done with a transesophageal probe (in other words, a tube that is inserted down the throat that the patient swallows) and shows the growths of bacteria on the heart valve and a blood culture that detects bacteria in the blood.

> If you know you have heart valve dysfunction, you will probably need to take antibiotics right before dental procedures (including teeth cleanings) and most types of surgery in order to prevent the chance of infection from the procedure traveling to your heart.

CARDIOMYOPATHY

Another reason for heart failure is damage to heart muscle cells that can be caused by a virus, some types of chemotherapy used to treat cancer, and sometimes pregnancy. The name for heart failure of this type is *cardiomyopathy*. In some instances the heart fully recovers from the disease or the effects of the drug or pregnancy, and in other instances the damage remains, but is manageable and does not progress. In some cases, however, the heart progresses to very severe heart failure. Heart failure medications can be effective in such cases, but in some patients the best chance of improvement is a heart transplant, or the implant of a partially mechanical heart device called a left ventricular assist device, or LVAD, to assist the patient's heart, until a donor becomes available for transplant.

HEART FAILURE

The reason I call heart failure the important "second face" of heart disease is that the number of deaths and hospital admissions for heart attacks have dropped in the last several years, while the number of deaths and hospital admissions for heart failure is going up. In fact, heart failure is now the most common diagnosis of patients being hospitalized with heart problems!

Heart failure is a condition in which our hearts either become weakened and pump blood less well, or become stiffer and less able to fill with blood between each heartbeat. The result of both of these conditions is the increased pressure of the blood in the heart, which in turn increases the pressure of the blood in the lungs, leading to increased shortness of breath during exercise, and in severe cases, even at rest. The pressure also causes fluid to leak out of the blood vessels in the legs and cause swelling. Heart failure is commonly the result of heart attacks, after which there is too little good muscle left in the left ventricle. Heart failure is also commonly caused by high blood pressure, which makes the left ventricle work harder against the pressure in the arteries. In addition to these two causes, damaged heart valves and diseased heart muscle (cardiomyopathy) account for a significant amount of heart failure.

Heart failure treatment is, in a sense, a new specialty area of cardiology, and cardiologists who now plan to focus their care on these patients often complete an extra year of training at a heart failure center. Medications, such as diuretics (water pills), digoxin, ACE inhibitors and beta-blockers, and, in some cases, Coumadin, can be very helpful in some patients, as can newer medications that are used for the same purpose. Studies have shown that exercise training will improve the symptoms in many heart failure patients without increasing their risk of a complication. Heart transplants, although very effective at reversing the symptoms of heart failure, are currently limited to people at the end stage of their disease, and then to only a small percentage of these people, since the supply of donor hearts is small and the incidence of heart failure is increasing.

Another important New Rules strategy is that if you have heart failure you should ask your cardiologist for a consultation with a heart failure specialist early in the disease, and then expect to be comanaged by your cardiologist and this specialist if the disease progresses and the symptoms increase. The skills, access to the latest drugs, and the access to procedures such as the implanted automatic defibrillators, left ventricular assist devices, special pacemakers, and transplants by a heart failure specialist can result in a heart failure patient living significantly better and longer!

REMEMBER: WHEN ALL IS SAID AND DONE, "TIMING IS EVERYTHING"

Outliving heart disease involves incorporating all of the steps or New Rules discussed in this book to address, prevent, and assess risk; detect heart disease if you have it; and, if indicated, obtain the best medical and lifestyle treatments to manage your disease. For many of us, however, these strategies, while necessary, will not be sufficient to prevent risky surgeries. Even by adhering to the best medical and lifestyle programs, at some point in our lives we may develop heart disease and learn, after the appropriate tests, that fixing the blood vessels with surgery or angioplasty is the only way to further prolong our lives and allow us to be symptom free. For many of my patients, especially those who have been active participants in my 92nd Street Y Cardiac Prevention Program, needing invasive steps seems at first to be a failure of the program. In fact, these invasive procedures are part of a successful program to outlive heart disease, since they allow us to live longer and better lives.

Armed with the information in this book regarding the latest science and clinical evidence, you can be an informed advocate for your own best care. Putting this information into practice is in a sense the art that complements your knowledge of the science. This art is the art of communication, the art of polite interrogation, and the art of being effectively assertive with your physicians. Your management of your condition will play an important role in all of the New Rules discussed here, but none more so than the issue of having the "best" tests for you and, if indicated, the best surgery, angioplasty, or other procedures at the right time, at the right place, performed by the right person.

UNDERSTAND THE CONNECTIONS AMONG YOUR GENDER, YOUR HERITAGE, AND HEART DISEASE

Throughout this book I've referred to the studies from which my colleagues and I have developed the protocols for the ways we treat heart disease, but there is a caveat—and it's an important one: most of these studies were performed on Caucasian men. As recently as 10 years ago, heart disease in women was thought to be a rarity, and there are still very few studies that include non-Caucasian populations.

The "GO RED" campaign of the American Heart Association and other national medical organizations has dramatically increased the awareness of heart disease risk among women in the United States. Today mentioning "women" and "heart disease" in the same breath isn't revolutionary, but it was before this campaign. Championed by women health care professionals, this movement has led us to look carefully at a woman's awareness of her risk, how women are viewed by physicians and the health care system, and the real information—or lack thereof—about risk factors, symptoms, and treatment. This new and

broader focus on women's health has resulted in better knowledge about heart disease before and after menopause, contra-
ception, and pregnancy, and the important differences between
men and women regarding risk factors, cardiac testing, treatment, surgery, balloon angioplasty, and the varying symptoms
experienced when a heart attack is occurring. Much of this
material has been presented in earlier chapters, but it is important to emphasize it again in one place. Even though the disease
is the same, there are differences in the ways it presents itself in
the two genders. There are also indications that various ethnic
groups experience heart disease onset and symptoms in different
ways and at earlier ages than the white males on which our
knowledge is based. The bottom line: If you are a woman or are
non-Caucasian, being aware of those differences can help you
outlive heart disease.

WOMEN AND HEART DISEASE: A REVIEW

As recently as a decade ago, many physicians presumed that
women were much less likely than men to have coronary artery
disease. Data from a large study that included EKG stress testing
and coronary angiograms showed that women with chest pain
and positive stress EKG tests were less likely than men with the
same symptoms to have disease-narrowed coronary arteries.
Then physicians looked at the data further and noted that
women were just as likely, or *more* likely, to die of cardiovascular disease than men; they just did so when they were about 10
years older than their male counterparts. Further studies showed
that women were diagnosed later and with more disease than
men, at least in part because physicians were less likely to look
for coronary artery disease in women and so less likely to order
the necessary tests to check for it. To make the issue even more

difficult, most of the large clinical trials up to that time had no (or very few) women enrolled, and thus the clinical importance to women of their findings was unknown.

The list of pertinent issues for women with regard to cardiovascular disease is growing each year. I have summarized below the items that are of most importance to your program to outlive heart disease:

1. Physicians, the general population, and (still) many women are unaware of the high risk of cardiovascular disease in women.

2. If you are a woman, you are more likely than a man to experience angina pectoris or a heart attack with "atypical" symptoms (including burning pain high in the abdomen, sharp pain in the chest, profound weakness, shortness of breath, and dizziness)—the "typical" symptoms being pressing or dull pain, which may travel to the left arm or neck. The real problem with this difference in the way you experience heart attack or angina pectoris is that both you and your doctor are less likely to think about heart disease when the symptoms are not "typical," that is, typical for a man, and, as we learned in New Rule No. 1, delay in getting treatment can limit your chances to outlive your heart disease.

3. While the risk factors for coronary heart disease and stroke are generally the same for women and men, there are important differences. These differences include the actual impact (how much each factor increases overall risk), how risk factors change with aging, and the value of specific risk-reduction treatments.

4. Some of the noninvasive tests to find coronary heart disease and, if present, to determine how severe it is,

are less accurate for you than they are for men. Having the right test at the right time is very important.

5. The benefits of coronary artery bypass surgery and angioplasty are, in some instances, less favorable for you than they are for men, due, in part, to the greater amount of heart disease and the older age at which you might undergo these procedures as compared to men. Decisions about angioplasty and surgery always require careful evaluation and thinking, but even more so if you are a woman!

In order to outlive heart disease, it is critically important that you are aware of your risk of developing and dying of coronary heart disease. The facts are sobering:

1. Heart disease is the major cause of death of women, with deaths from cardiovascular disease being more than twice those due to cancer.
2. One in eight women aged 45 to 65, and one in three women over the age of 65, have clinical evidence of cardiovascular disease.
3. If you are an African American woman, your risk is even greater—two-thirds higher than the risk for your Caucasian counterparts.

In order to win the battle against cardiovascular disease, you need to be aware of your risk factors and important differences regarding these risk factors and their clinical symptoms of heart disease. This awareness is especially important, given the information lag about women's health among some practicing physicians and emergency medical center staff.

HOW YOUR GENDER AFFECTS YOUR HEART DISEASE RISK FACTORS

Although atherosclerosis looks the same in everyone's blood vessels and can result in similar damage to the heart muscle and other organs, there are real differences in the way you may experience the onset of a heart attack and the way men do. The way men experience heart attack has been mentioned elsewhere (see New Rule No. 1, beginning on page 17), and you may also experience these "typical" symptoms. However, you may also experience "atypical" symptoms outlined below:

1. For women, your first sign of coronary heart disease is most often angina pectoris, whereas for men it is a heart attack. It is important to note that if you have heart disease, you will be less likely to experience the pressing chest pain during angina that a man typically does. Instead, you will more often experience symptoms such as burning pain in the middle-low chest to high-stomach area, often confused with indigestion or heartburn; or profound weakness, sweating, and dizziness. The opportunity to intervene before a heart attack damages heart muscle requires that you seek prompt medical attention for these symptoms and that your doctor is aware of the real possibility that they represent coronary artery atherosclerosis.

2. Emergency approaches to interrupting a heart attack by administering a clot-busting drug in the emergency room or taking the patient quickly to a cardiac laboratory and opening the artery work equally well in both genders. But if you show up in an emergency room, you may be less likely to be fast-tracked with procedures to detect that you may be having a heart

attack, due to your "atypical symptoms" and a lack of
"gender awareness" on the part emergency room staff.
Immediate and repeat EKGs and blood tests for heart
attack are essential to making this diagnosis in time to
open the artery and save important heart muscle. Given
this situation, it is clear that you must, if you are to
win the battle against heart disease, go quickly to an
emergency room when you experience typical or
atypical symptoms and be assertive about getting
immediate testing for a heart attack. Also, since many
(in fact, most) visits will not result from a heart
attack, but may be a dangerous form of angina
pectoris called "unstable coronary syndrome," it
might be wise of you to ask about having a stress test
before going home, or in the next few days. The stress
test, often done with echo- or nuclear imaging, is the
best way of separating those at high risk for unstable
coronary syndrome (who have high likelihood of
having a cardiac event over the next six months)
from those of you without evidence of this syndrome
(who can safely be sent home to set up a scheduled
appointment with your doctor). Even when there are
borderline EKG changes and mild elevations in the
blood test for a heart attack, a prompt coronary
angiogram is often indicated.

3. Your lipids profile, which has been stable or even
   improving as you age, will worsen, and your blood
   pressure will rise as you enter menopause and will
   continue in this direction as you continue in the
   postmenopausal period of your life, all of which
   increase risk of a heart attack. This is in contrast to
   men, in whom the rise in lipids and blood pressure is
   more gradual. The strategy here is to start a New

Rules diet and exercise program as you approach menopause (if you haven't already done this) and to have your blood lipid levels checked twice a year if they are normal. Have your blood pressure checked more frequently than twice a year if it is borderline. Many women will benefit from drugs such as statins for their lipids and treatment of elevated blood pressure. Diabetes also becomes much more likely as you pass through menopause and beyond, and testing for this disease at your annual and then twice-a-year lipid measurements is a very good idea.

SPECIAL RISK FACTORS FOR WOMEN

If you are a woman, see New Rule No. 2, beginning on page 26, for a discussion of general risk factors that apply to you. Below, I want to emphasize that certain risk factors for heart disease are even riskier for you—and explain why.

Smoking

Cigarette smoking in women represents an increased risk of developing heart disease, even when set against comparable smoking by men. Smoking has decreased in the United States since 1965 (the peak recorded incidence of smoking in this country), but far more so among men than among women. This fact, combined with the fact that young men and women are equally likely to start smoking, has resulted in a near-equal, by gender, incidence of smoking. The impact of this rise in the number of women smokers is seen from the results of the Nurses Health Study, mentioned several times in earlier chapters. Women who smoked a pack or more of cigarettes a day had a fivefold increase in risk of coronary heart disease and myocardial infarction when compared to nonsmoking women. The basis for the marked increase in coronary heart disease in smokers as compared to nonsmokers is only partially understood. Men and women smokers both have an increase in cholesterol and triglycerides compared to nonsmokers, and smokers of both genders are more insulin resistant and oxidize more LDL cholesterol than nonsmokers, but *the increase in heart attack risk is greater, per cigarette smoked, for women than for men!*

Passive smoke exposure at home and in the work place has been the focus of recent studies. The results are surprising. Living with a smoker or working in a location where people smoke is associated with an increased risk of heart disease. Studies of blood platelet and endothelial function show sharp turns for the worse when we are exposed to secondhand smoke.

The New Rules about women, smoking, and outliving heart disease are obvious:

- If you smoke, try *repeatedly* to stop. People who have succeeded in stopping have tried an average of nine times before finally quitting and not smoking for over one year. In the Nurses Health Study, women who had stopped smoking had a 30 percent lower risk of heart disease after two years, compared with women who continued to smoke! Smoking cessation in women has been associated with weight gain—and a return to smoking. Diet and exercise programs to prevent weight gain, therefore, play an important role when you are trying to quit smoking.
- Be assertive about your right to live and work in a smoke-free environment. The laws in many states now protect this right, so forcing others to comply with the law will save many lives—and lower your own risk of heart disease.
- Do everything you can to prevent your children from start-

ing to smoke. You are fighting powerful and insidious prosmoking forces, but winning this battle for your children is one of the best gifts you can give them. Write, call, speak out against, and boycott companies and institutions that actively or passively support smoking.

Physical Activity

Studies of women (Nurses Health Studies and others) have shown a reduced incidence of heart disease in active versus sedentary women: this incidence is reduced in relation to the amount of activity (more is better!). A study of men and women who engaged in an exercise program after a heart attack showed that, with regard to changes in HDL, women were at an advantage. HDL cholesterol increased initially in both genders, but after one year it was still increased only in women. Exercise, as demonstrated in clinical studies, can reduce the postmenopausal adverse changes in cholesterol lipoproteins. It thus is an essential part of heart-healthy living for you and a rule for outliving heart disease.

Diabetes

This is the most "gender-different" risk factor for women when compared with men. Women with diabetes have a risk of developing heart disease that is five times that of nondiabetic women, and their threefold increase in risk of a heart attack is greater than the twofold risk experienced by diabetic men. Your chance of developing diabetes increases significantly after menopause; an increase in your fasting blood glucose level after menopause is a powerful predictor of this risk. The likelihood that you will develop diabetes if you have a fasting glucose level over 130mg/dl *doubles* when compared to women who have lower level. The increased risk of heart attacks in diabetic women is due both to the diabetes itself and to the increased likelihood of having high blood pressure and of being overweight if you are diabetic. The combination of these risk factors, called metabolic syndrome, dramatically raises your chance of having a heart attack. If you have this syndrome, take steps outlined in previous New Rules chapters to correct it.

THE "NEW" RISK FACTORS FOR WOMEN

C-Reactive Protein

This is one of the "new" risk factors (see New Rule No. 2, beginning on page 26), but data from recent studies have indicated that it may predict a heart attack even in women with low LDL cholesterol. CRP is considered a marker of the inflammation that plays such an important role in atherosclerosis. It is produced in the liver in response to chemicals that rise during inflammation in the arteries. In the Women's Health Initiative study, completed in 2005, an elevated CRP was a stronger predictor of heart disease than was LDL cholesterol, causing almost a threefold increase in heart events during the first three years of the study. Statins reduce CRP, presumably, by inhibiting the inflammation process. This effect occurs very early—within two weeks of starting the drugs. In contrast to the effect of statins on LDL cholesterol, CRP reduction using a statin is not a dose-response effect. Increasing doses of statins in men and women did not bring CPR down to a lower level when compared with the usual starting doses.

Homocysteine

In a recent study of men and women in Europe, and in the Nurses Health Study in Boston, an elevated blood level of homocysteine, a substance your body makes as it uses the amino acid methionine, was found to increase the risk of a heart attack, stroke, and other arterial disease to almost the same extent as cholesterol and smoking. The increase in risk with each rise in the blood levels was in fact slightly greater for women than it was for the men in the study. An important finding was a very strong association of high blood pressure in people with high blood homocysteine levels. If you have elevated homocysteine, make sure to check your blood pressure frequently. Elevated homocysteine can be reduced by taking folic acid with B6 and B12 vitamins and, until very recently, this was standard therapy. However, the recently completed NOVIT trial, presented at the European Society of Cardiology Congress in 2005, looked at the effect of treating heart attack patients with folic acid, B6, or both. This study has changed the thinking with regard to folic acid supplements for elevated homocysteine. Folic acid lowered homocysteine, but did not reduce second heart attacks or strokes, and when folic acid and B6 were taken together, the second heart attack rate increased by 20 percent. Women can discuss taking folic acid (alone) with their doctor if they have high homocysteine levels in their blood, but should not take folic acid and B6 together.

Lp(a)

This is a two-part lipoprotein molecule in the same family as LDL cholesterol, but with an important difference. One component acts enough like LDL cholesterol to promote atherosclerosis. The other component acts enough like an enzyme called plasmin that our bodies produce to rapidly dissolve early blood clots and thus help prevent heart attacks. This component can compete with our own plasmin and also increase our risk of a heart attack. Several studies have shown that an increase in Lp(a) is associated with an increase in heart attack risk, and one study showed this was true in older women. High levels of Lp(a) are mostly due to our genes and not our lifestyle. We have no really effective drug to lower Lp(a); niacin works to a moderate degree, but is not widely used because of its side effects (skin flushing, itching, and stomach discomfort in many people). The answer is to lower all of your other risk factors. If you have high Lp(a), you should lower your LDL cholesterol and aggressively address all your other risk factors.

HOW YOUR GENDER MAY AFFECT NONINVASIVE TESTING FOR CORONARY ARTERY DISEASE

As we discussed in the "best tests" section (New Rule No. 8, page 165) of this book, noninvasive testing may be performed for two reasons:

- to detect significant narrowing of one or more coronary arteries of the heart (coronary heart disease detection), and
- to help estimate your risk of a heart attack (coronary heart disease risk assessment).

If you are a woman, exercise EKG testing alone is less accurate in detecting heart disease, especially if you are premenopausal, than it is in men, partly because of a lower likelihood that premenopausal women with symptoms will have heart disease than will a man of comparable age and symptoms. This phenomenon—that a test will be less accurate when used in a population in which the disease is found in only a small percentage of the people (heart disease in 40- to 55-year-old women) than in a population in which it is more prevalent (men of the same age)—is very real, although not easy to understand. It is referred to as Bayes Theorem, discussed earlier in the New Rules chapter on risk. Another theory, not yet proved, to explain this phenomenon has to do with a differing biological response of the heart's blood vessels and muscle cells during exercise in premenopausal women as compared with that of men of the same age.

Because of this phenomenon predicted by Bayes Theorum, you will likely have a stress test (if you need one) that uses nuclear- or echocardiogram imaging to improve the accuracy of the test. If this test leaves the presence or absence of coronary artery disease in doubt, your doctor may recommend that you undergo a coronary angiogram or have a CT angiogram, if this procedure is available.

One value of exercise stress EKG testing that is not diminished in women, especially if you are postmenopausal, is its ability to accurately assess your risk of having a heart attack over the next several years. This is especially true when equations developed from studies of women are used to estimate the risk. One such system, the Duke Treadmill Test Score for women, has been well studied and should be part of the final interpretation of your stress EKG test.

THE RISK AND CLINICAL VALUE OF ANGIOPLASTY/ STENTING AND CORONARY ARTERY BYPASS SURGERY IN WOMEN

Coronary artery bypass surgery has, until recently, been thought riskier for you than for men. Early studies showed that women had more complications and a greater risk of death during or after the surgery than did men. We now realize that this difference is due, in large part, to the fact that you are usually diagnosed later in your disease and at an older age than are men, and are more advanced in your heart disease than the average male patient undergoing the same surgery. In 2003 a study of more than 2,000 patients who had CABG surgery in the United States showed higher death rates among women, but when other disease factors that would increase the risk of surgery were considered, gender alone was not associated with higher CABG surgery death rates. In carefully studied and evaluated women, the value and the risk of CABG surgery is no different for you than it is for a comparably compromised man.

The clear message here is that your individual risk factor of a serious complication or death with CABG surgery should be an important consideration in deciding in favor of, or against, this surgery, as it is with a man. Your gender alone should not be the basis of this decision!

The stenting findings have gone in much the same direction as the CABG findings with regard to women. The early studies showed a higher rate of complications following angioplasty in women. When, however, the older age and the higher prevalence of diabetes and other conditions in the women patients were considered in a National Institutes of Health study of procedures performed in the United States, the conclusion was that gender was not a predictor of recurrent heart attack or death while a patient was in the hospital for the procedure, or during a one-year period following the angioplasty. What made the difference was the woman's general health before the invasive procedure.

Bottom line: Being a woman should *not* be the basis of a decision against undergoing coronary artery bypass surgery or angioplasty when these procedures are clearly indicated by symptoms and coronary angiography! The outcomes in otherwise healthy women will match the success rate of men.

A SUMMARY OF YOUR NEW RULES RISK FACTORS FOR HEART DISEASE

Seek immediate medical attention for chest pain or other acute and distressing symptoms such as stomach or chest burning, shortness of breath, dizziness, or weakness. Be aware that some physicians and other medical personnel may still not address the issue of heart attack or heart disease unless you specifically and assertively address this matter with them. Make sure you get a prompt EKG and blood tests for cardiac markers when (not *if!*) you go to an emergency facility for the above symptoms.

See your physician for recurrent symptoms, both typical and atypical, and discuss risk factors and the value of noninvasive testing. This testing is critical, since the medical establishment may not appreciate your risk for heart disease!

Monitor your cholesterol profile (LDL, HDL, triglycerides, and total cholesterol) every two years in the years prior to menopause and at least every year thereafter. Remember: a good profile before menopause in no guarantee of a good profile after menopause.

Monitor fasting blood sugar levels every year, after menopause. Higher values (over 130mg/dl) reflect a significantly increased risk of developing diabetes. Place special emphasis on reducing body weight, controling blood pressure, and avoiding smoking, if your blood sugar is rising.

Monitor your blood pressure and initiate treatment with your physician if your reading is over 139/89. Treatment should lower your reading to 139/89 if you do not have heart disease, diabetes, or multiple risk factors, and to below 135/85 if you have these risk factors, or others. Remember that "prehypertension" is a blood pressure reading above 135/85 but below 140/90. If you are in this range you should start a DASH diet and engage in a regular exercise program. Also, you and your doctor should aggressively lower all your other heart disease risk factors.

Start a New Rules–type diet as early in life as you can, but especially as you approach menopause. Calculate your BMI and pay attention to body weight and work to reduce calories, if indicated.

Start a regular exercise program, especially as you approach or enter menopause. This, along with other risk-factor reductions, will lower your overall risk and attenuate the increased risk for heart disease associated with menopause.

AFRICAN AMERICANS AND HEART DISEASE

The success rate to date in the prevention and treatment of heart disease if you are African American has lagged behind that of Caucasian Americans. In the data available as of 1996, the death rates from cardiovascular disease (mostly heart attack and strokes) were about 50 percent higher for black men as compared to white men, and almost two-thirds higher for black women as compared to white women. In part this increase in death rate is due to socioeconomic issues and their impact on risk factors, and to health care disparities. There are, however, important biological issues that must be addressed, if you are African American, in order to outlive heart disease.

These biological issues are no doubt due to genetic factors shared by many African Americans. In the near future we will be able to produce a meaningful analysis of an individual's genetic makeup, and know which risk factors are the most important and which drugs will have the best and the worst impact on your health. At the moment, we have to use the crude observations of patterns identified in your immediate family or shared by a significant number of people of a specific race in order to find common genetic factors that are important with regard to heart disease.

In general terms, the impact of heart disease risk factors is nearly the same across all races. That means that risk factors such as a high LDL cholesterol or elevated blood pressure will increase risk to about the same degree in all races and both genders. The initial Framingham group was essentially all Caucasian, but in recent studies, African American families from a nearby community have been enrolled in the study to address the issues of racial differences. *If you are African American, you need to pay very close attention to high blood pressure and diabetes.*

High blood pressure is more prevalent, may be more difficult to treat, and its impact on heart attacks and strokes is greater for you than for people of other races. The data are chilling, to say the least. Three studies have noted that very high blood pressure, over 180/110, is two to three times more prevalent in African Americans than in whites, and that the death rates from conditions related to high blood pressure were three times higher in African Americans. A study that is somewhat dated, but no doubt still correct, noted that African American men under age 45 are *10 times more likely to die of complications of high blood pressure* than are white men of the same age. Diabetes is 50 percent more prevalent in African Americans than in white Americans, and African Americans with diabetes are more than twice as likely as their white counterparts to also have high blood pressure that is untreated or poorly controlled.

The impact of these findings on the New Rules program to outlive heart disease for you, if you are African American, is to increase the focus on lowering high blood pressure and monitoring for diabetes, and to know the impact of these conditions on your risk of having a heart attack or stroke.

STRATEGIES FOR AFRICAN AMERICANS REGARDING BLOOD PRESSURE AND DIABETES

High Blood Pressure

Prevent or delay the onset of high blood pressure by taking the following steps:

- Start eating the DASH diet modified for high blood pressure to reduce salt intake, as discussed in New Rule No. 5, beginning on page 96. This diet is an essential strategy for you and for your entire family!
- Start a program of regular exercise as outlined in the New Rule No. 4, beginning on page 73, and encourage your family to join you. During family time, look for active family activities instead of passive activities (such as watching TV).
- Work continually on keeping or reducing your weight to a healthy level, ideally at a BMI of 25 or less. Maintaining a BMI that low is not easy, but it is very important to come as close as you can to a BMI of less than 25.

Detect high blood pressure as soon as possible after it occurs. Check your blood pressure and that of each member of your family twice a year from age 12 onward, and follow up any borderline (over 135/85) or high (over 140/90) values with repeat blood pressure measurements within two weeks!

Get early and effective treatment for high blood pressure, if you develop it.

- Although it is tempting to try diet, weight reduction, and exercise to lower blood pressure, especially if your levels are only slightly over 140/90, it is likely that you will need medications as well. (With your doctor's advice, you can always reduce or stop medications as your blood pressure comes down with diet and exercise.) In many cases, a single medication will not be effective, and two or more medications will be required. The point is to get your blood pressure down and keep it down. The number of medications or doses is not the important issue. The lower blood pressure reading is!

• Be aware of side effects and report them promptly to your doctor. If you are going to stay on medications to keep your blood pressure in a normal range, then you need those medications that produce no, or very few and mild, side effects in you. If you suffer side effects, the chances are that you will probably stop taking your meds and suffer the more serious consequences associated with high blood pressure. Work with your doctor to find a medication or combination of medications that can be taken once a day *in the morning,* which will also increase the likelihood that you will stay on the treatment. Remember that you will be on medications to reduce blood pressure for the rest of your life. The goal is to make your life a long and healthy one, not to take fewer medications.

• Buy and use a home blood pressure machine, write down your readings, and bring your records to your doctor at each visit.

• Monitor kidney function with periodic blood and urine tests at your doctor's office. Heart attacks and strokes are only two of the major diseases that are brought on by high blood pressure. Kidney failure, especially if you are African American, is the third.

Lower all the other modifiable risk factors to lower your overall risk of a heart attack or stroke. High blood pressure is an important reason to stop smoking, lower LDL cholesterol to below 100 (preferably below 70), and keep your weight down!

Diabetes

In most instances, what is termed adult-onset diabetes results from the cells of our body becoming resistant to the effects of our own insulin, thus making it necessary to raise the amount of insulin secreted into our blood by our pancreas. Eventually, the pancreas can't keep up with this increased secretion demand, and our blood sugar will then increase. In many cases we treat elevated blood sugar levels with pills, but in some instances injections of insulin are required. The other type of diabetes, juvenile diabetes, most often occurs in childhood or adolescence and is the result of the failure of the pancreas to produce insulin. Here, injections of insulin are the only effective treatment.

If you are African American, you are at risk of developing diabetes. Here are some rules to prevent it.

Prevent or delay onset of diabetes.

- Reducing or keeping your weight at a good level—at or below a BMI of 25—is even more important in preventing diabetes than it is for preventing high blood pressure. The epidemic of obesity in the United States is the major reason for the epidemic of diabetes and will be, if not controlled, the reason for increasing disability and death from heart attacks and stroke.
- Weight loss and an exercise program will delay and in some cases prevent the onset of diabetes if you have metabolic syndrome.

Detect diabetes as soon as possible.

• Have your fasting blood sugar measured at each annual visit to the doctor. If it is already borderline or if you meet the list of criteria for metabolic syndrome, consider having your blood tested twice a year after age 30. If it is borderline or high, expect to be sent for a glucose tolerance test, which measures blood sugar by a blood test every hour for four to five hours after drinking a special high-sugar drink, and another blood test called a Hemoglobin A1C. This test measures the amount of hemoglobin that has been chemically altered by the sugar in your blood. Because this is a slow process, your level of Hemoglobin A1C reflects your average blood sugar in the preceding 30 days.

• If you find yourself urinating more frequently, or if you have infections in your urinary tract that make you feel the urge to urinate more and cause some burning and pain during urination, see your doctor promptly. These symptoms are often the first sign of diabetes.

Get early and effective treatment for diabetes, if you develop it.

• Studies now clearly show that keeping your sugar in a good range for as much of the day as possible will result in less damage to your blood vessels and your kidneys, and will reduce your risk of a heart attack or stroke. The marker of this level of blood-sugar control during the past month is the level of Hemoglobin A1C in our blood. Good treatment will keep this level below 7.

• Expect to be placed on two types of pills to control diabetes. Remember that the goal is control, not pill counting!

Know your overall risk for heart disease. This New Rule is even more important if you are African American since, by the time you develop full-blown adult-onset diabetes, you probably will have been insulin-resistant for several years, and we now understand that this state of insulin resistance promotes atherosclerosis. In other words, by the time you become diabetic, you probably already have coronary artery atherosclerosis. We treat diabetic patients as if they are secondary prevention patients— that is, patients who already have coronary artery disease. Thus, in order to outlive heart disease, it is mandatory to lower LDL cholesterol to 70 instead of 100, reduce blood pressure to below 135/85 instead of 140/90, and address every other risk factor for heart disease. These matters are even more critical for you, because diabetes is more prevalent in African Americans than in the general population.

HISPANIC AMERICANS AND HEART DISEASE

If you are Hispanic American, you know that this term refers to a diverse group that includes people of Mexican heritage (the largest group by far in the United States, making up 60 percent of all Hispanic Americans), Cubans (16 percent, predominantly living in the Southeast), Puerto Ricans (living in the Northeast), and other Caribbean, Central and South American Latinos. You have a broad diversity in core ancestry, and we've discovered that cardiac risk profiles differ among these populations. Thus, it is probably not reasonable to apply findings in one group to others. Those of you who are of Mexican ancestry, as you would expect from your numbers, are the most studied in the United States with regard to heart disease.

In general, heart disease risk factors and their impact are the same as those noted in non-Hispanic whites, with the exception of the consistent finding that, as a Mexican American, you have an increased risk of developing Type 2 (adult-onset) diabetes, which is related in part to the increase in obesity among Hispanic men and women, compared with non-Hispanic whites and blacks. This difference is especially true among women, in whom the prevalence of diabetes is more than twice that found in non-Hispanic white women.

Since the onset of diabetes is related in large part to obesity and inactivity, there is a clear need for you to emphasize the importance of diet (especially with regard to the amount of calories that are eaten every day) and physical activity. In terms of diagnosis and treatment of diabetes, it is clear that early diagnosis, with good blood sugar control and aggressive cholesterol-lowering and, if needed, blood pressure–lowering treatments, are of great importance to you.

The plan that offers the best chances in this regard is the one outlined in the section addressed to African Americans, who share this same increased risk of developing diabetes. The strategies of prevention, early detection, effective treatment, and overall risk-factor reduction noted above are critical parts of a New Rules program to outlive heart disease for you and, although we don't have good data to tell us this, most probably for other Hispanic American populations as well.

ASIAN AMERICAN POPULATIONS: JAPANESE, CHINESE, AND SOUTH ASIANS

Japanese

If you are Japanese American, the fact that today you have about the same likelihood of developing heart disease as do Caucasian Americans tells us something about the importance of lifestyles issues when compared to genetic factors in preventing heart disease. In 1958, the first year of the Seven Countries Study, Japanese people living in Japan had the lowest rate of heart disease death among the countries studied, due no doubt to their diet, which was lowest in fat and cholesterol, and a lifestyle that was extremely active. The Ni-Hon-San study looked at diet, blood cholesterol levels, and heart disease death rates of Japanese in Japan, those who had migrated to Hawaii, and those who were living in the United States (mostly in San Francisco). The heart disease rates in Japan have remained very low, although they have increased as the amount of fat in the Japanese diet has increased; the rates in Hawaii were higher and the diet more typically Western; and the heart attack death rates for people of Japanese ancestry who were born in the United States were the highest, and the same as those of the general U.S. population. We are what we eat, and we are how we live. For you as Japanese Americans, the lesson is clear: a heart-healthy diet and exercise program are critical issues to outliving heart disease, and all of the New Rule strategies apply!

Chinese

If you are Chinese American, good information specific to Chinese Americans regarding the risk factors for heart disease is surprisingly sparse. What we have, in the way of information about heart disease in China, addresses risk factors and heart disease death rates of people living in the country's rural provinces versus in the urban areas. This data show that all of the standard risk factors, such as cholesterol, high blood pressure, obesity, and inactivity, are considerably worse in people living in urban areas. Very limited data is available regarding Chinese people living in the United States. In one 10-year-old study of a cholesterol-screening project in Chinatown in New York City, the cholesterol levels were higher than those in urban areas of China and in fact were comparable to a group of non-Chinese Americans screened as a part of this project. Even without good studies, it is reasonable to think that you are subject to the same lifestyle risk factors that affect all Americans, and that you will require the same attention to diet, exercise, smoking cessation, and cholesterol to lower your risk. Thus, the same New Rules attention to symptoms, risk assessment, and the best testing and treatments apply to you as to others who want to outlive heart disease.

South Asians

South Asian communities in the United States have often retained the cultural, dietary, and social patterns of your homeland, and then have tended to marry within their own groups. Those of you of Indian ancestry from Guiana, South America, fit this description and have the same increased risk of heart attack and cardiac death. This risk is so significant that the 1996 edition of the respected *Oxford Textbook of Medicine* includes Asian race, most notably South Asian, as an atherosclerosis risk factor.

My colleagues who are of Indian ancestry are very much aware of this risk; some of them are also my patients. I first became aware of the incidence of heart attack in the Guiana Indian community, however, when I was conducting rounds at the Brooklyn Hospital Center's coronary unit. The resident presented a case of a 43-year-old taxicab driver who had emigrated from Guiana and had come to the emergency room with a burning pain high in his abdomen. He did not smoke, was slender, had only slightly elevated blood pressure, and his EKG was normal. In my discussion with the residents, I wondered aloud why he was admitted to the hospital, much less the coronary care unit; the senior resident told me that being of Indian ancestry from Guiana was, in this hospital's experience, a strong marker of cardiac risk. Later that day I was told the result of the patient's angiogram—severe disease of all three of the heart arteries. He was sent for CABG surgery the next day.

In the last 20 years, India has seen a dramatic rise in death due to coronary heart disease and stroke, and an associated rise, most pronounced in cities, in high blood pressure, cholesterol, and smoking. The prevalence of heart disease is especially high in expatriate communities of Indians, as reflected in data from the 1980s that show a 40 percent higher heart disease death rate in South Asians living in England and Wales as compared to the general population. Studies conducted in India showed that the standard risk factors, including diet, obesity, diabetes, and physical inactivity, as well as cholesterol, high blood pressure, and cigarette smoking, explained in large part this rise in heart disease. These and other studies suggested that insulin resistance, an important aspect of the metabolic syndrome, may play a role in this high heart disease mortality rate. Some of the high heart attack rate in India and in Indian communities in other countries is probably related to a vegetarian diet that is often high in saturated milk fats.

The issues are not yet fully understood, but what is clear is that Asian Indians in India and in other countries have a rising rate of heart disease that is higher than the populations of almost every other country, and that the major risk factors, especially diet-related obesity, insulin resistance, high cholesterol, and high blood pressure, are the basis for most, if not all, of this increase.

Therefore, if you are South Asian, you should embrace a program of prevention with risk factor reduction, early detection, and optimal treatment from an early age, and be especially ardent at engaging in regular physical activity and maintaining a BMI under 25. You should embark on a New Rules program at an early age to prevent heart disease and to outlive it, and as an essential part of living long and living well.

SUMMARY POINTS: GENDER, HERITAGE, AND HEART DISEASE

- Women are more likely to die of heart disease than men because they experience "atypical" symptoms and are usually diagnosed at a later stage of the progression of their disease.
- Women should demand careful screening and analysis of their "atypical" symptoms when they are seen in an emergency room.
- Women who smoke have a greater risk *per cigarette* of having a heart attack than do men.
- Elevated CRP level in women is a stronger predictor of heart disease than elevated LDL cholesterol levels.
- A woman's risk of complications following heart surgery is no greater than that of a man who has a similar stage of disease.
- African Americans' death rate from cardiovascular disease is 50 percent higher than that of Caucasian men, and nearly two-thirds higher than Caucasian women.
- High blood pressure—a significant risk factor for heart disease—is more prevalent in African Americans and more difficult to treat in African Americans than in Caucasians.
- Hispanic Americans are a diverse group and some are at greater risk of developing heart disease than Caucasians, although the data are sketchy as to specifics. There is increased prevalence of diabetes.
- Asian American populations have an increased risk as compared to their Caucasian counterparts of developing heart disease, probably due in part to genetic factors.

PARTNER WITH YOUR DOCTOR TO REACH YOUR HEART-HEALTH GOALS

My advice to transform you and your doctor into a dynamic duo involves more than merely having a nice relationship with a medical professional. In most cases, this is relatively easy to establish, since you share the same general goals. My advice is about becoming an informed, knowledgeable partner with your physician so that both of you are aware of the most important issues to address as well as the pitfalls that might prevent you from getting the best heart-health care.

PATIENT COMPLIANCE VS. PHYSICIAN COMPLIANCE: A NEW RULES PERSPECTIVE

Some of the questions that I frequently encounter when I preach this doctrine of informed partnership to groups of cardiac patients and their families are:

- Why is it necessary to be an informed, assertive health care partner with my doctor? Why can't I just trust my doctor, follow his or her advice, take my medications, and be confident that I am getting the best care?
- How do I become informed without being "pushy" and, if I am informed, am I sending a message that I don't trust the doctor?

The first question is a totally reasonable one, and it is only in the past five years that I have come to understand how important it is. Study after study of physician practices with regard to heart disease prevention and treatment reveal a very important flaw. *Good doctors fail in one-third of their patients or more to treat cholesterol and blood pressure to the guideline-recommended levels.* These are the levels that the most recent scientific studies have shown to reduce fully your chances of having a heart attack. Of equal concern is that good doctors *frequently* do not use all of the important drugs that have been demonstrated to be effective and important in reducing your risk of a heart attack. Missing out on the protection of these drugs means that you are being denied the best chance of beating heart disease! Equally damaging to your best chance of outliving heart disease is that good doctors will, in the *majority of patients,* commonly not provide direct and useful counsel regarding diet, exercise, and smoking cessation when it is clearly required.

This issue has a name, "physician compliance with evidence-based guidelines," and the American Heart Association, fully aware of the problem, has initiated a major national program for doctors called "Get with the Guidelines."

I was recently invited to participate in a National Institutes of Health (NIH) Special Emphasis Panel that reviewed grants addressing this problem. Strategies to improve guideline compliance ranged from reeducating physicians, using office staff to follow treatment responses, and my favorite—an electronic medical record that compares the patient's treatment to guidelines on the doctor's computer screen at each visit, which blinks in red when there are discrepancies. A recent article in a major medical journal, by clinical investigators at Emory University in Atlanta, rang true to my ears. They proposed that the failure of physicians to treat lipids, blood pressure, and diabetes to guideline levels is due to what they termed the doctor's clinical inertia–failure and suggested reasons why this occurred. The electronic record will, I think, in the future be an effective solution to this problem, but for now patients need a quick and effective fix. I strongly believe that the only effective fix is an informed patient who knows what the treatment levels regarding cholesterol and blood pressure should be, and who makes sure the doctor helps him or her reach them.

Dr. Thomas Pearson, who received his NIH Preventive Cardiology Academic award in the same year that I did, designed a project to measure, in a group of 5,000 patients with high LDL cholesterol, how many patients achieved the guideline treatment levels. The findings were very scary! In this group of 5,000 patients with high LDL cholesterol, guideline levels were reached in less than one in four patients at low cardiac risk, less than one in three patients at intermediate risk, and in less than one in five of the patients at high risk or with heart disease!

Women fared even worse. Doctors from the University of Iowa compared LDL guideline levels to LDL cholesterol levels in women with known heart disease who were considering joining a study of the effect of estrogen and progesterone hormones on heart disease. Despite the fact that they all had heart disease, fewer than half were on statins and fewer than one in ten was at the guideline level (100mg/dl) for patients with heart disease.

The story with high blood pressure is no better. Here we have excellent information from the large, federally funded National

Health and Nutrition Examination Surveys (NHANES). Data for the last study, NHANES III, reveal that only two-thirds of those surveyed with high blood pressure knew that they had it, only about one-half of these patients were being treated, and less than one in four patients was found to have guideline levels of BP (less than 140/90) at the time of the survey. Some of these findings are attributed to the reluctance on the part of doctors to treat systolic, or "top number"–only high blood pressure, despite the recent clinical evidence that doing so will significantly prevent heart attacks and strokes.

Armed with this knowledge, the answer to the question "How do I get the best care?" is now obvious. You are going to get the best care from your doctor only if you know what best care entails, and if you monitor it. To do so, you need to inform your doctor that you intend to be an involved partner who will work effectively with him or her in obtaining the best care the doctor can provide.

CHOOSING A DOCTOR

The following is a list of important things to consider when selecting your doctor and, when necessary, your cardiologist. Although this list may seem to state the obvious, you would be surprised how often one or more of these standards is not met.

Nature of the Doctor's Practice:

1. *Does the doctor practice* in a group that provides night and weekend emergency coverage, or as a solo practitioner who has coverage provided by other well-established and qualified physicians? A group practice is usually preferable to the coverage arrangement.
2. *Does the doctor have a front office staff that is available,*

will work with you to schedule tests or procedures, will make sure that your doctor calls you back within a reasonable time frame, and will schedule you promptly when you have symptoms or complaints that are of concern?

3. *Is the doctor affiliated with the best hospitals in your community?* It is important that the physician is affiliated, where possible, with a hospital that performs cardiac surgery and coronary angioplasty. A full-service cardiac hospital will also perform diagnostic exercise EKG testing, provide nuclear- and echocardiography testing with a dedicated staff, and have additional services, such as an electrophysiology service, that provide advanced diagnostic testing and treatment of patients with arrhythmias.

4. *Does the doctor have a person dedicated to handling billing procedures?* This would be a person who is available to help you sort out the very frequent problems that come up with your health insurance or managed care company. I never realized how important this service was until a family member had an injury that required diagnostic testing, surgery, and rehabilitation. The physician's offices had a billing manager with whom I could speak that saved me hours on the phone. While billing procedures shouldn't be linked to quality health care, they are part of the reality we deal with in the age of managed care, and will certainly be an aspect of patient satisfaction.

Training and Personality of the Doctor

1. *Is the doctor "board certified"* in primary care (family practice or internal medicine) or cardiology? "Board

certified" means that your doctor has completed a quality-monitored residency-training program, has been recommended by the physician faculty of this program, and has passed a written examination prepared by a board of highly qualified specialists in the field. Although some doctors who are not board certified are excellent, and some with board certification are not, this credential is a good place to begin when selecting your doctor.

2. *Does your physician have the right personality* to work with an informed patient? Here is where the partnership issue will succeed or fail. The physician who believes that he or she is the expert whose care you have sought and whose judgment you should not discuss (much less question) is not going to be a good partner. If a doctor gives you the impression that your questions regarding his advice are the same thing as questioning his judgment, and further suggests that you should seek another doctor if you continue, that doctor is right! You should seek another doctor! A less arrogant but equally dysfunctional attitude is what I call the "Marcus Welby" model, in which the doctor doesn't challenge you but displays a "father-knows-best" attitude that limits discussion and gently implies that all you need to do is listen to the sage advice (and be quiet and passive). I try to instill in my cardiology fellows-in-training that they do well to welcome questions, view their role as that of a patient-educator, and provide clear information. But the most important role a doctor can perform is to listen, listen, listen! Most of my patients, some with prodding on my part, assume the role of informed partners who want to address the basis for important decisions.

When they perform this role, hopefully they can
understand my reasons for the drugs, tests, or
procedures that I am recommending and how I am
prioritizing the issues of greatest importance to *them*.
This focus is a key component of "best care."

Very often, you won't actually choose your cardiologist, especially when you seek a referral from your primary care doctor.
Two things you can do to make sure you get a true health partner: (1) Ask your primary care physician to recommend a cardiologist who will consider you a partner in your health care. (2)
Tell the cardiologist at your initial consultation how highly you
value doctors who are open and informative, and who view the
patient as a partner.

Important Patient Services

1. Does the cardiologist's office *ensure that you'll receive
   copies of the results* of blood tests, EKGs, and other
   important studies, such as coronary angiograms and
   angioplasty procedures? These documents should be in
   your home file and you should let the doctor know you
   will be asking the office staff for copies of these reports.
2. Will the cardiologist provide a *copy of your latest
   EKG* for you to carry in your wallet or purse? This
   information, plus a list of your medications, allergies
   to drugs, major procedures or surgeries (type and
   date), and a statement regarding your heart diagnosis
   (for example "high blood pressure being treated, high
   LDL cholesterol being treated") is essential. Among
   the first rules of outliving heart disease is to go to a
   hospital emergency room immediately if you have
   chest pain, get an EKG, and compare it with the last

one you had. Having these critical parts of your medical history on hand will help you obtain the most immediate and effective care.

THE INFORMED AND ASSERTIVE PATIENT CHECKLIST

Here is the list of concerns that should be discussed with your doctor and should be monitored by you. I have added some background material to the list so that you can use it effectively. Also, since it's not a bad idea to carry this list with you on your first several visits, I also have included a brief take-along version.

A First Step—Know Your Risk

1. First, know your risk: If you do not have heart disease you should have your risk estimated as (circle one) LOW—INTERMEDIATE—HIGH.
2. If you have diabetes, have had a stroke, or have peripheral vascular disease, and if you have a high risk (*over* 20 percent chance of a heart attack in the next 10 years), you should be managed with regard to medications and goal levels of *cholesterol and BP as if you have heart disease.*

Educate Yourself about Drug Treatment

Although some of this information is presented in several New Rules chapters, I am including a summary of the drugs that we know, based on strong clinical evidence, prevent heart attacks in people without heart disease (primary prevention) and in people who already have coronary heart disease (secondary prevention).

Aspirin (primary and secondary prevention)

If you have had a heart attack, or are a man at moderate-to-high 10-year risk of a heart attack, you should, in most cases, be taking an 81mg aspirin (one-quarter of a regular aspirin) every day. People with increased risk of bleeding, or those who have had bleeding stomach ulcers or bleeding into the brain, should not take aspirin. Data from four major trials in men conducted over the past 20 years show that first and second heart attacks are reduced by more than 25 percent with just one 81mg pill a day! In a large study of women, only those who had had a heart attack did better on a daily aspirin. There was no value in taking aspirin to reduce the chance of a heart attack, and thus only risk, for women with increased risk factors but no history of a heart attack. But there was a reduction in stroke. Thus, taking aspirin if you are a woman without heart disease is a discussion you need to have with your doctor. Further studies will, no doubt, address the value of aspirin in women at very high risk who do not have heart disease, but at present this question remains unanswered. Since there is a small risk of serious bleeding, aspirin should not be given to men at low risk according to the Framingham tables (see New Rule No. 2, beginning on page 10). Full-dose aspirin has a somewhat higher risk profile. From the studies, an equally protective effect is achieved from the quarter-strength aspirin.

Note: It is thought that one of the ways aspirin staves off heart attacks is by preventing the formation of early clots that involve our platelets. Recent studies have indicated that about one in ten of us is aspirin-resistant, meaning that aspirin will not block our platelets from becoming activated to form clots. A urine test can identify such people while they are taking aspirin, and studies under way may, in the near future, identify people for whom aspirin isn't working and for whom an alternative drug such as clopridogrel (Plavix) would be of value. We do not have the data yet, but ask your doctor about this test at least once a year.

Beta-Blockers (primary prevention only)

If you have had a heart attack, you should in most instances be on a beta-blocker such as propranolol (Inderal), metoprolol (Lopressor), or atenolol (Tenormin). Studies from the United States and Europe have shown that after a heart attack, beta-blockers reduce your risk of dying by more than 25 percent. There is, however, no evidence that beta-blockers will help reduce chances of a first heart attack in patients who are at increased risk of heart disease; *you should, in general, not take this medication only for this purpose.* Since, however, beta-blockers are often used to treat high blood pressure and arrhythmias (irregularities in your heartbeat such as atrial fibrillation—see below), patients who have not had a heart attack will often have this drug appropriately prescribed for high blood pressure or abnormal heart rhythm.

Statins or other cholesterol-lowering drugs (primary and secondary prevention)

These drugs reduce heart attack rates by more than one-third in people without heart disease and in those with heart disease. The following material summarizes the levels of the cholesterol and blood pressure that you should have with or without treatment. (See New Rule No. 3, beginning on page 58, about taking statins.) I usually give my patients this list after their first blood tests and strongly encourage them to discuss any medications listed, including those that I have not prescribed. I also encourage them to ask for their blood pressure and blood cholesterol results after every blood test so that they can compare them to the guideline numbers.

The desirable levels for cholesterol are different for different people depending on your 10-year heart attack risk. Low risk of a heart event is less than 6 events in 100 people over 10 years, intermediate risk is between 6 and 20 events in 100 people over 10 years, and high risk is more than 20 events in people over 10 years. The "one-minute" scoring sheets for men and women below will tell you in which category you fit (remember that as you get older, even without risk factors, your 10-year risk goes up) and which are the levels that will give you the best chance of outliving heart disease.

Your Risk	Desirable Level of LDL cholesterol
Low risk	less than 160
Intermediate risk	less than 130
High risk	less than 100*

* In many instances your doctor will decide to use the much lower number of 70.

If you haven't already calculated your risk, and don't want to turn back in the book for a complete explanation, the committee of experts that chose these goals presented a simple method of estimating your risk for the purpose of cholesterol treatment. Risk factors for choosing your desirable cholesterol numbers according to the cholesterol guidelines include:

• High blood pressure (either top or bottom number over 140/90)
• Obesity
• Sedentary lifestyle
• Cigarette smoking within the last five years
• High LDL, low HDL,* or high triglycerides[†]

*Below 40 for a man and 50 for a women
[†] Above 150

If you have 0–1 risk factors, use the **low-risk** numbers. If you have 2 or more, use the **intermediate-risk** category.

If you have coronary heart disease or diabetes, peripheral vascular disease, carotid artery disease or have had a stroke, use the **high-risk** numbers. Also if you have the metabolic syndrome, use the high-risk numbers.

If you need to be treated to lower your cholesterol, which means you are above the guideline numbers, or have good numbers but have had a heart attack, angioplasty, surgery, or are being treated with drugs for heart disease, you should expect to be treated with one or more of the following types of drugs. (If not, ask why not!)

1. *Statins:* (simvastatin [Zocor], pravastatin [Pravachol], atorvastatin [Lipitor], fluvastatin [Lescol], lovastatin [Mevacor], rosuvastatin [Crestor]. These once-a-day pills are the first choice for high LDL cholesterol and have, as our New Rule No. 3 indicates, "rewritten the rules" for outliving heart disease. There is a small chance of side effects that include muscle pain or soreness, most often felt in the upper legs or arms, and an increase, above normal, in one or more liver tests. These numbers revert to normal when the statin is stopped. There is a very slim chance (less than one in a million) that a patient could have a catastrophic complication of toxic breakdown of the muscle cells, which would lead to kidney failure, which can be fatal. Kidney failure is most often seen when two types of cholesterol drugs are used together (statins + fibrates [such as Lopid or Tricor—see below] or niacin). Even

in these instances, the risk is very low and is far outweighed by the better chance of living longer that is afforded by the drug combination. Careful monitoring by blood testing can help to reduce this risk.

2. *Fibric acid drugs:* There are two drugs in this class: fenofibrate (Tricor) and gemfibrazil (Lopid): Both lower LDL cholesterol, although less well than the statins, but they increase HDL and lower triglycerides much better than the statins. If you have a reaction to the statins (muscle pain, liver inflammation), then these drugs are the next-best choice to lower LDL cholesterol, and if you have low HDL or high triglycerides alone or as part of the metabolic syndrome, these are first-choice drugs. Combining them with statins will, as I noted above, increase very slightly the chance of the dangerous muscle breakdown syndrome. Clinical studies suggest that this complication is seen less with Tricor than with Lopid.

3. *Niacin:* A very effective "drug" at 1 to 3 grams a day to raise HDL and lower triglycerides. It will also enlarge the size of LDL cholesterol particles to a point that we think is less dangerous. It is referred to as a drug, not as a vitamin, since the dose we use is 20 to 50 times the amount contained in a vitamin pill.

4. *Ezetimibe (Zetia):* This drug is very effective when combined with a statin to increase the drop in LDL cholesterol. It is not associated with muscle pain or the dangerous breakdown of muscle cells. When used by itself, it is a modest reducer of LDL cholesterol.

5. *Bile acid resins:* These are the oldest of the cholesterol drugs we have. They cause us to lose bile acids in our feces so that our body uses cholesterol to make more

bile acids. Used rarely and usually in combination with other cholesterol drugs, this drug's most common side effects are constipation and "gas."

There are two other classes of drugs to ask your doctor about.

Angiotensin Converting Enzyme Inhibitors (often referred to as ACE inhibitors) and Angiotensin Receptor Blockers: These drugs stop the production or block the effect of Angiotensin II—a stress-related hormone —on the heart, blood vessels, and kidneys. They are very effective drugs to lower blood pressure, and have been shown to help protect the kidneys in patients with diabetes. A large study called the HOPE trial (for Heart Outcome Prevention Evaluation) demonstrated that adding the ACE-inhibitor Ramipril to a statin in people with elevated cholesterol only (in other words, they did not need the Ramapril to lower blood pressure) lowered the rate of heart attack deaths. As a result of this study, I often add Ramipril to a statin in patients with elevated cholesterol. You and your doctor should discuss this.

Hypertension Drugs: If you have high blood pressure, you should be treated with medications as well as with a salt-reduced DASH diet and an exercise program. Treating high blood pressure to "safe" levels is essential to outliving heart disease. The levels of blood pressure that require treatment and the current guideline levels you should be treated to are summarized below. Another important thing to do: buy and use a home blood pressure–measuring device. Bring the device you purchase with you on your next visit to your doctor's office so that the readings can be compared with your office readings. It is important that the two readings be very close in order to be sure that your home device readings are accurate. Discuss with your doctor how often and when during the day you should measure your blood pressure at home.

BP Classification	Systolic (top number)	Diastolic (bottom number)
Normal	below 120	below 80
Pre-hypertension	120–139	80–89
Stage 1 Hypertension	140–159	90–99
Stage 2 Hypertension (greater risk)	over 160	over 100

Pre-hypertension is not a disease, but it does mean that you will probably develop real hypertension (Stage 1) over time. Diet (DASH) and exercise are very important if you fall into this category. The treatment goal for Stage 1 and Stage 2 hypertension is below 140/90, unless you also have diabetes or kidney disease, in which case the goal is below 130/80. Monitor your blood pressure at home and in the doctor's office; if your readings do not meet guideline goals above, discuss the matter with your doctor. In most instances, increasing the dose of a medication you are currently taking, or adding an additional medication to your treatment will be his or her response. Commonly used medications include diuretics (water pills), beta-blockers (discussed earlier), ACE inhibitors (also discussed earlier), calcium channel blockers such as amlodipine (Norvasc), diltiazam (Cardiazam), or verapamil (Calan), and angiotensin-receptor blockers. A variety of additional drugs are also commonly used, and can be very effective.

ESSENTIAL LIFESTYLE TREATMENTS TO PREVENT FIRST OR SECOND HEART ATTACKS

Lifestyle changes are not just "good things to do." They are medical treatments and should be discussed with your doctor. As noted below and elsewhere in this book, ask for referrals to a registered dietician and to a cardiac rehabilitation program, if you are eligible. These professional services are of enormous value, and well worth the persistence and assertiveness that it might take to get them!

Diet

The only real-world diet demonstrated to reduce heart attacks is the Mediterranean diet, supplemented by fish or fish oil capsules, as used in the Lyon Heart Study. The DASH diet I use in the New Rules plan is a modification of this diet. This diet includes at least eight servings of fruits and vegetables; moderate-size meat, poultry, and fish portions; and whole grain breads and pastas. If your doctor doesn't mention the Mediterranean/DASH diet, you should. You should also ask for your weight and height to calculate your BMI (see chart in New Rule No. 5 on diet, beginning on page 96).

Although you can begin eating a Mediterranean /DASH diet on your own, your doctor can be a big help by giving you a prescription to meet with a registered dietician. The prescription will allow you to contact your medical insurance or managed care company for dieticians who participate in your plan, and schedule an appointment to start to modify your diet, a great first step toward outliving heart disease. The New Rule No. 5 on diet also offers you a good way to get started.

Exercise Program

Exercise is a critical part of a program to prevent heart disease, and to outlive it if you already have it. If you have heart disease (a heart attack, angioplasty, CABG, or a diagnosis of angina pectoris) ask you doctor to refer you to a cardiac rehabilitation program. This is the best way to begin the right kind of exercise and also to get excellent information on diet. Studies show that heart patients who engage in such a program after a heart attack have a 15 percent reduction in heart attack deaths. Your doctor can also order or perform a valuable exercise EKG stress test to determine the point at which you would usually stop due to exhaustion, fatigue, or symptoms. This test will provide you with a maximum heart rate that can be used in training and, more important, give you the confidence that you can exercise safely!

State of Mind Issues

As discussed in New Rule No. 6 beginning on page 118, depression represents a real risk for having a first or second heart attack, or for dying of heart disease. Take the simple test for depression in that chapter. If your score indicates depression, talk about it with your doctor, ask for a referral to a mental health specialist, and start exercising. Therapy, group programs, or medications may provide relief. Consider all the options. Also, if you are isolated, try to reestablish important relationships with your friends and family. Studies suggest that building social support acts to counter the risk of depression and anxiety.

Here is the simple, take-along form of the checklist:

DOCTOR'S VISIT CHECKLIST

If you do not have heart disease you should have your risk estimated as (circle one) (LOW) – (INTERMEDIATE) – (HIGH) – (HAVE HEART DISEASE or Heart Disease equivalents).

MEDICATIONS

Aspirin: (always *unless contraindicated* by allergy or bleeding if you have heart disease, and almost always if no heart disease but risk is intermediate or high)

Dose____(81mg probably best)

Statin or other cholesterol drugs if your LDL cholesterol is high for your 10-year risk level

Now: (__/__/__) Total Chol_____   LDL Chol _____
HDL Chol_____   Trig_____

Evidence-based goal levels: Chol_____   LDL_____
HDL_____   Trig_____

Metabolic syndrome: NO   YES

Medication(s) and dose:_____

_____

Beta-Blocker:

Had a heart attack or unstable coronary syndromes? YES NO

Medication(s) and dose:_____

_____

ACE Inhibitor:

Have abnormal lipids requiring treatment? YES   NO

Medication (Ramipril or other) and dose:_____

_____

BLOOD PRESSURE

BP today ___/___/___/ Evidence-based BP target levels: 140/90–130/80

Medication(s) and dose:_____

_____

DIET: Ask for referral to Registered Dietician.

EXERCISE: If heart attack, angioplasty, or CABG surgery, or angina pectoris: Ask for referral to a cardiac rehabilitation program: _____ AND ask for exercise EKG examination (with or without nuclear- or echo-imaging)_____.

STATE OF MIND: If you score as depressed on the scale in New Rule No. 6, Understand the Mind-Body Connection, beginning on page 118, if you feel down or hopeless, talk with your doctor about depression and ask for referral_____.

SUPPLEMENTS: If you have heart disease, ask about fish oil capsules (1 to 2 grams a day).

IT ALL ABOUT THE DETAILS

A rule of scientific experimentation that I learned from my Chief of Cardiology, Dr. Norman Krasnow, during my training was that the devil is in the details. This maxim is even more true of outliving heart disease. Along with an excellent program of prevention and treatment, you need to be tested for conditions that can cause you to have a stroke, a lethal heart irregularity, or a spontaneous rupture of a major artery with massive bleeding. The following are the recommended tests. They are important in order to lower as much as possible the chances of these sudden events happening.

Carotid Artery Ultrasound Testing

Sound waves are used to generate other sound waves that bounce back from the tissue in the carotid arteries, the major arteries to the brain. The bounced-back (echo) signals are processed to provide a picture of the arteries and estimate the degree of obstructive plaques that may be found there and in other arteries. Plaques that fracture and form clots that break off and travel to the brain are the cause of most strokes. The presence of a very large plaque that blocks 90 percent of the inside of the arteries, or lesser plaques that block more the 70 percent of the artery but occur in a person with symptoms of TIAs (transient ischemic attacks, or prestrokes), is a reason to consider surgery or stenting of the arteries. Although there is risk of stroke from the stenting procedure itself, these treatments will significantly lower your risk of a stroke. For most of us, few things are more important.

I order this test when my patients reach age 65—or earlier if they have heart disease, develop symptoms, or I hear a sound over the arteries with my stethoscope.

Abdominal Ultrasound to Evaluate the Abdominal Aorta

The same echo technique as described above is used to create a picture of the aorta, the large artery in the back of your abdomen that carries the blood from the heart. This test looks for a ballooning out of part of the vessel. If this ballooning is present and if the size of the area is half again as large as the regular vessel, there is a real risk of a rupture with massive bleeding and death. Early detection of this process, followed by stenting of the aorta or surgery, will prevent rupture—and add years to your life. The ballooning is due to atherosclerosis and all the major risk factors for developing heart disease (abnormal lipids, high blood pressure, and smoking) are among the factors that further increase your risk.

I order this test at age 60 to 65 in all my patients—earlier in men and if there is heart disease or stroke, or if they have increased risk factors, especially smoking.

Atrial Fibrillation

As we age, the chance increases that the chambers on the top of our heart, called the atria, will replace their normal pattern of contracting and relaxing with a condition in which thousands of areas of the atrial wall contract and relax independently. The result is that the atrium quivers, a condition known as atrial fibrillation. This condition often causes a fast and irregular heartbeat, as impulses are showered down at random on the conducting pathways to the lower ventricles. The fast rate is usually easily slowed with medications, but the quivering atria have created an area where early blood clots—called thrombi—can form. These thrombi can then break off and travel with the blood to the brain—to cause a stroke. The risk of this happening with atrial fibrillation in people over 70 years old or with any heart abnormality is about 5 in 100 patients a year, which is quite high! Treatment with a drug that reduces the formation of thrombi in the blood, called Coumadin, will reduce this risk to near that of a person with a normal heart rhythm. The drug must be carefully monitored with a blood test and most of my patients have such a blood test each month. In 2005 the FDA approved home testing kits, similar to the blood sugar kits that people with diabetes use. These kits can make the monitoring process safer and easier.

Detection is the major concern with atrial fibrillation, because the condition is easy to miss. Many people could not sense a fast or irregular heart beat before they had a stroke. Thus a person with atrial fibrillation may not see a doctor or have it detected, and may not be placed on Coumadin. Knowing if you have atrial fibrillation is therefore a critical New Rule to avoid a stroke. There are two strategies that can help.

1. Each year I ask all my patients at risk of atrial fibrillation (over 70, or with heart problems) to wear a "Holter Monitor" (the size of a small portable cassette tape recorder and first mentioned in New Rule No. 8), which records their EKGs for 48 hours. A computer scans these tapes looking for any abnormal rhythm—in this case, atrial fibrillation.
2. I teach my patients to take their pulses and have them do it with me so that they appreciate how a regular pulse feels. I ask them to check their pulses for one minute every week, and if one of them feels an irregular pulse, to come in to see me right away. This simple test will help you to detect atrial fibrillation early enough to make a definite diagnosis and start treatment to reduce to the lowest degree possible your subsequent risk of a stroke.

SUMMING UP: THE CRITICAL DOCTOR-PATIENT PARTNERSHIP

One last word about your part of the partnership: *Being informed and assertive is critical to getting best care, but so is following the advice your doctor gives, which involves being conscientious enough to take all your pills at the right time, or near the right time, every day.* If this parting advice sounds too silly to bother to mention, remember the reality is that we all lead very busy lives and find it very difficult to adhere to "pill schedules." Also, as the number of pills we take and the number of times a day we are required to take them increases, the chances are less that we will take them and get the full value of our medications. When I discuss this fact with medical students, their first reaction is that the patients who don't adhere to doctors' instructions don't understand how important they are, or don't care. Then I ask them a simple question: "How many of you who have been treated for a sore throat with an antibiotic took the pills every day for the full 7 or 10 days, as prescribed?" The show of hands in the classroom is always very small. Once the throat pain is gone they stopped taking their pills, despite understanding the importance of the full course of therapy in completely eradicating the infection!

When I ask myself the same question, I do no better, although I am now diligent (probably missing only one day every two weeks) about taking my statin, aspirin, and fish oil capsules. The rules are simple: Try to work with your doctor to take all your pills in the morning. If you must take a pill two or three times a day, try to leave a supply where you will be, and try to link in your mind taking the pills with a usual activity such as lunch, dinner, or preparing to go to sleep. Don't be surprised if you have trouble with this instruction. I am sure your doctor would as well—but keep trying. Your ability to outlive your heart disease may depend on it.

Glossary

ADENOSINE TRIPHOSPHATE (**ATP**)   A high-energy substance, produced when muscle cells metabolize sugars and fats. It is the fuel that is used for the body's physical work and functions.

ALPHA LINOLENIC ACID   The vegetable form of omega-3 fatty acids, found in flaxseed or canola oil. See FATS.

ANGINA PECTORIS   Chest pain, usually brought on by exercise or stress that may indicate that a coronary artery is blocked by greater than 70 percent by atherosclerotic plaque.

ANGIOGRAM   A test in which a coronary artery is injected with a substance that shows up on an X-ray and provides a picture of the inside of that artery. Used to detect atherosclerosis (plaque formation) in the artery.

ANTIOXIDANTS   A class of chemicals found in foods that may help prevent or stop atherosclerosis, since the chemicals may serve to inhibit an early stage of the disease that involves the oxidation of LDL cholesterol.

APCS (ATRIAL PREMATURE CONTRACTIONS) AND VPCS (VENTRICULAR PREMATURE CONTRACTIONS) occur occasionally in all of us and usually do no harm. Recurring extra heartbeats that arise in the atria can result in a fast rhythm that often requires treatment. Of greater concern is a period of continued extra heartbeats that arise in the lower part of the heart, the ventricles. These extra beats can cause symptoms and in some cases may be a harbinger of ventricular fibrillation, which, if not interrupted, will lead quickly to death. *See* NORMAL SINUS RHYTHM.

ARRHYTHMIA   A changed pattern of heartbeats caused by an interruption to the electrical signal that regulates them. Arrhythmias can be stopped or stalled beats, or a slow heart rate, or long pauses that occur between beats. Arrhythmias can also be "extra" heartbeats, or groups of extra heartbeats.

ATHEROSCLEROSIS   A complicated multistep process by which blood vessels become occluded with plaque, reducing blood flow to vital organs such as the heart and brain. Atherosclerosis can be the cause, when a plaque's surface is broken, of an early clot, called a thrombus, which blocks the coronary artery (and causes a heart attack) or breaks off and plugs an artery to the brain (and causes a stroke).

AUTONOMIC NERVOUS SYSTEM   Also called the involuntary nervous system and consists of the sympathetic and opposite-acting parasympathetic (or vagal) nervous systems.

BAYES THEORUM   A mathematical theory, named after the Anglican priest in England who described and proved it, that says that the ability of an imperfect test to correctly detect or exclude a finding (for instance, coronary artery disease) is determined in part by the likelihood of the finding (coronary disease) in the population tested. That is, the more likely a person is to have heart disease, the more accurate the test will be in detecting or excluding it.

BLOOD PRESSURE   The amount of force that blood exerts against the walls of arteries. This pressure is measured in millimeters of mercury, since the gauges that doctors used to use contained a thin tube partially filled with mercury. We now recognize the danger of mercury to the individual and the environment, so the gauges use other techniques to measure the pressure. When the heart is pumping more blood into the arteries, blood pressure rises. This highest value is called the systolic blood pressure. When the heartbeat is concluded and blood is not being pumped into the arteries, the blood runs off into our muscles and organs and the pressure drops. This lowest pressure is the diastolic pressure. If the pressure is higher than 140 systolic or 90 diastolic, it is high blood pressure, also called hypertension.

BODY MASS INDEX (**BMI**)   A calculation that relates a person's height to weight to determine whether or not he or she is underweight, over-weight, or obese. BMI is calculated using metric system units (height in meters divided by weight in kilograms squared). Another way to cal-culate BMI using inches and pounds is BMI=(weight in pounds divided by height in inches squared) x 703. A better way to learn your BMI is to look at a table that has height in inches and weight in pounds. A BMI above 25 indicates overweight and over 30 indicates obesity.

CAD   Acronym for coronary artery disease, commonly referred to as heart disease, when the arteries become blocked by cholesterol and other material called plaque. CAD is the reason for 98 percent of all heart attacks.

CARBOHYDRATES   Sugars, either simple or complex, found in food. Simple sugars are found in fruit juices, some vegetables, honey and maple syrup, and table sugar. They are usually rapidly absorbed across the walls of our intestines and increase the glucose concentration in our blood. Complex carbohydrates are found in vegetables and whole fruits, and require further metabolic breakdown in our digestive sys-tem before we can absorb them. They cause our blood sugar to rise more slowly. Carbohydrates produce 4 calories per gram, should make up 50 to 60 percent of total calorie consumption, and should come mostly from complex carbohydrates from foods like vegetables, whole grains, and fresh fruits, as opposed to the simple sugars in soda, candy, or syrups, or from starches such as potatoes.

CARDIOMYOPATHY   Damage and weakening of heart muscle cells that can be caused by a virus, some types of chemotherapy, and sometimes other conditions, such as pregnancy, that can lead to heart failure.

CAROTID INTIMAL MEDIAL THICKNESS MEASUREMENT BY ULTRASOUND The process of atherosclerosis takes place in the intimal layer of the wall of the artery, between the most inside endothelial cells and the adjacent medial layer of smooth muscle cells. Measuring the thickness of this intimal layer in the wall of the artery by ultrasound is a measurement of the degree of atherosclerosis. Since atherosclerosis is a diffuse process and this measurement is in the carotid artery of the neck (which is close to the skin and thus easily measured by ultrasound with a high degree of accuracy), this test reflects the overall extent of plaque development in an individual. This test does not measure specific plaques, but in most instances the greater the carotid-medial thickness, the more likely the patient is to have many and large plaques in the coronary arteries.

CENTRAL OBESITY   A waist measurement greater than 40 inches in men or 35 inches in women that reflects the buildup of fat below the skin of our abdomen (our "stomachs") and inside, around our intestines. This fat buildup is often a telltale sign of high heart attack risk called the metabolic syndrome.

CEREBRAL-PITUITARY-ADRENAL AXIS   A term that refers to the brain's control of the release of hormones, such as adrenaline and cortisone, by the adrenal glands that respond to stress. This mechanism is used every day by the brain to alter the biological system for day (active stress) and night (safe rest). This axis is a critical part of the body's response to injury and stress, helping, among other things, to expand our blood volume and increase the activity of our platelets to form clots. Overuse of the mechanism in response to constant stress and production of cortisol (as seen with depression) will accelerate atherosclerosis and increase the risk of heart attack.

CHD   Acronym for coronary heart disease, used to refer to the major form of heart disease—atherosclerosis of the arteries of the heart. Only late in the disease, when the diseased arteries cause the heart muscle cells to be deprived of oxygen-rich blood, is the heart muscle itself involved.

CHELATION THERAPY   A process that involves the infusion, via a catheter placed in an arm vein, of a solution that contains the substance EDTA and vitamin C, selected B vitamins, and magnesium. EDTA, an accepted treatment for lead poisoning, will bind to heavy metals in the blood, including calcium, and cause them to be excreted in our urine. When we thought that removing calcium from the plaques of diseased arteries would make them shrink, chelation therapy made some (even if very little) sense. Now that we know that the calcium is not removed and the procedure has no effect on plaque, chelation is definitely not recommended for heart patients.

CHOLESTEROL   A molecule that the body uses for multiple purposes, including lining the membranes around cells and as a building block for hormones and other substances essential to life. "Cholesterol" when used as a generic term refers to the group of particles of cholesterol and fats that travel in the bloodstream. These particles are both absorbed in the bloodstream as we digest our food and manufactured by the liver and circulated by our bloodstream. One form of cholesterol, called LDL (for low-density lipoprotein) cholesterol, is found, usually in large amounts, in atherosclerotic plaques in the arteries.

CHOLESTEROL PROFILE   A blood test that should be taken every two years in men and women and at least every year in women after menopause to measure LDL and HDL cholesterol levels, total cholesterol, and triglycerides.

COMPLEMENTARY MEDICINE   Alternative therapies, including herbs and vitamin supplements, homeopathic remedies, and specific treatments not utilized and often not recognized to be of value by traditional Western medical science. Complementary medicine products and treatments are, however, used by two-thirds of Americans at some point in their lives.

CORONARY ANGIOGRAPHY   A test that provides a high-quality X-ray picture of the inside of the coronary arteries. A hollow catheter, thinner than a drinking straw, is placed, via a needle puncture, into the femoral artery (the large artery at the top of the leg), and then advanced up through the main artery of the body, the aorta, until it reaches the opening of the two main coronary arteries. Here, a clear solution containing iodine that shows up on X-rays is injected into these arteries to produce a high-quality picture of the lumen, the inside opening, of the coronary arteries.

CORONARY ARTERIES   The arteries that supply blood to the heart muscle.

CORONARY ARTERY BYPASS GRAFT (CABG) SURGERY A major surgical procedure, using the mammary artery or a vein from the leg (the saphenous vein), whose purpose is to create a "bypass" around a very large atherosclerotic plaque that is blocking the coronary artery. The bypass increases blood flow to heart muscle and in many patients reduces the chance of dying from a heart attack.

CORONARY-PRONE EMOTIONS Another behavioral (as opposed to biological or physiological) mechanism that seems to increase heart attack risk. These emotions include anger, hostility, depression, or anxiety. *See* CEREBRAL-PITUITARY-ADRENAL AXIS.

COUMADIN A drug that reduces the clotting process in the blood. It is used in all patients who have their heart valves replaced with mechanical valves by surgery and in most patients who have the arrhythmia atrial fibrillation to prevent a stroke.

C-REACTIVE PROTEIN (CRP) A protein that indicates inflammation in the body and in the wall of the arteries due to atherosclerosis. CRP predicts the likelihood of coronary artery disease in much the same manner as do elevated cholesterol levels.

CYTOKINES Small hormonelike substances released by cells, especially when there is inflammation, as in atherosclerosis. When LDL is oxidized, cytokines are released in the wall of the artery that attract even more LDL cholesterol and white blood cells into the arterial wall to form plaque.

DASH DIET A Mediterranean-style diet, originally developed to control high blood pressure, but now thought to be the basis of the best, tastiest, and most balanced eating plan for almost everyone. The DASH diet grew out of a diet intervention study called the Dietary Approaches to Stop Hypertension study. It was developed to lower blood pressure in those patients who were suffering from hypertension.

DEFIBRILLATOR A device that delivers an electrical charge to heart muscle that is beating irregularly to stop the arrhythmia that is a threat to the person's life.

DEPRESSION Persistent and prolonged feelings of sadness, futility, and fatigue. Depression is a powerful predictor of the development of cardiac disease and heart attacks in otherwise healthy people. Depression is thought to alter the balance of the sympathetic and parasympathetic nervous systems to increase heart attack risk, and is one factor likely to contribute to the death of patients who have heart disease.

DIABETES MELLITUS   A condition that occurs in two different forms. Most diabetes that affects adults is known as type II or adult onset diabetes. In type II diabetes, the body becomes resistant to its own insulin and therefore has to overproduce insulin to try to keep blood sugar levels within normal range. Type I or juvenile diabetes occurs when the cells in the pancreas that produce insulin are damaged and produce too little insulin. Type I diabetes always requires injections of insulin. Type II diabetes can often be treated with pills or a combination of pills and insulin.

DIASTOLIC BLOOD PRESSURE   *See* HIGH BLOOD PRESSURE.

DUKE TREADMILL INDEX   A formula, developed at Duke University, that factors in how long a patient exercises, chest pain during exercise, and presence of ST segment depression on the exercise EKG that will predict, with reasonable accuracy, a patient's chances of dying of heart disease in the next 10 years.

DYSLIPIDEMIA   Another term for risk-increasing cholesterol levels in the blood.

ELECTROCARDIOGRAM (EKG)   A test that measures the electrical impulses produced as the heart beats. The EKG is the best test to detect arrhythmias (abnormal beating of the heart). It is also the first test used in the emergency room to determine if a patient is having a heart attack or has had a heart attack in the past. Heart-wall thickening or enlargement of the left ventricular chamber due to high blood pressure or damaged heart valves or heart muscle can also be diagnosed from the EKG.

ELECTRON BEAM COMPUTERIZED TOMOGRAPHIC IMAGING OF CORONARY ARTERY CALCIUM (OFTEN REFERRED TO AS EBCT)   A calcium detection technique performed with a Computerized Tomographic X-ray machine, often a specific type of CT machine called an electron beam

CT. This machine produces a picture so fast that it "stops the heart" in motion (like a picture of a racehorse taken with a very short exposure time). Calcium in the heart wall shows up as bright white spots in the picture, and this calcium nearly always is due to atherosclerotic plaques in the walls of the coronary arteries. The test cannot determine how large each plaque is, but more calcium, measured as a higher calcium score, means more atherosclerosis in the coronary arteries, and an increased risk of a heart attack.

EXERCISE EKG TESTING   Oldest of the noninvasive tests used to detect atherosclerotic narrowing of the heart arteries, in which a patient's EKG is measured during increasing levels of treadmill or bicycle exercise until the patient is near exhaustion, has chest pain, or has a change in their EKG reading. If the coronary arteries are narrowed, then the heart muscle won't get all the blood it needs during exercise and this condition will show up as chest pain and a change in the EKG called ST segment depression.

EXERCISE ECHOCARDIOGRAPHY   Echocardiography that uses high-frequency sound waves to produce "echos," or sound waves, that bounce back from the different parts of the heart, in much in the same ways that ships at sea use sonar to map the ocean floor. The result is pictures of the moving heart, including the chamber walls and the valves between the chambers. Echocardiography, specifically a technique called color Doppler, also shows the direction and speed of blood flow within the heart.

EXERCISE STRESS NUCLEAR IMAGING   An exercise EKG test that involves an injection of a nuclear isotope to get a picture of the heart at peak exercise and at rest. (The isotope used originally was thallium and the test is now often referred to as a thallium stress test.) This test can also be performed by substituting an intravenous drug, such as persantine or adenosine, for the exercise. An area of the heart muscle supplied by a significantly narrowed coronary artery will pick up less isotope during exercise, and thus emit fewer gamma rays producing "cold spots" on the images of the heart that are produced.

FATS   Chains of fatty acids that are the richest source of energy, producing nine calories per gram. When the carbon atoms that make up the fat molecules are tied together by single bonds (one bond between each pair of carbon atoms) that fat is called "saturated." When some of these bonds are double bonds (two bonds between each pair of carbon atoms) the fat is called "unsaturated." A fat with all single-bonded carbons except for one double-bonded carbon pair is called "monounsaturated." Total dietary fat consumption, measured as a percentage of the total number of calories eaten each day, should be at or below 30 percent. Less than 10 percent of total calories (about one-third of our fats) should be saturated fats and the remainder should be mono- and polyunsaturated fats. Omega-3 oils from fish oil and the vegetable form of omega 3, alpha linolenic acid from flaxseed or canola oil, should be part of every diet.

FIBER   An essential dietary nutrient. The American Heart Association diets recommend 15 to 30 grams of fiber from food each day, about twice the amount in the average American diet. Fiber from oats, beans, or phylum (a bulk laxative powder) is characterized as soluble fiber (which will lower LDL cholesterol) and fiber from most fruits and vegetables is called insoluble fiber. The food servings that will achieve this recommended fiber amount include whole grain products, fruits or vegetables, and one serving of beans each day. Other good sources of soluble fiber include legumes, beans, and dried peas. Fruits, vegetables, and barley are a source of both types of fiber.

FREE RADICALS   Waste products from food metabolized in the body that may be responsible for the inflammation of plaque in our blood vessels. It is thought that inflammation causes the plaque to become unstable, rupture, and lead to heart attack.

HDL   High-density lipoprotein, also known as "good" cholesterol, is "cardioprotective" and inversely related to the risk of suffering a heart attack, that is, the higher a person's blood level of HDL cholesterol, the lower is their risk.

HEART FAILURE   A condition in which the heart either becomes weakened and pumps blood less well, or becomes stiffer and less able to fill with blood between each heartbeat. Both conditions increase the pressure of the blood in the heart, which in turn increases the pressure of the blood in the lungs, leading to shortness of breath during exercise

and, in severe cases, at rest. The pressure also causes fluid to leak out
of the blood vessels in the legs and cause swelling. Heart failure is
commonly the result of heart attacks when there is too little good
muscle left in the left ventricle and is also commonly caused by high
blood pressure and damaged heart valves, which make the left ventricle work harder to pump blood.

HEART VALVE DISEASE   Heart disease or heart failure caused by
mechanical problems, not plaque buildup. The most common valve
problems fit into two categories: (1) calcified stenosis of the aortic
valve and (2) degenerative mitral valve insufficiency. Less common, but
not infrequent valve disorders include mitral stenosis (the mitral valve
doesn't open completely) and aortic insufficiency (the aortic valve
doesn't close completely and therefore leaks).

HIGH BLOOD PRESSURE   Also called hypertension, an increase above a
healthy level of the pressure that is in the blood of our arteries. The
highest pressure achieved, usually at the peak of the ejection of blood,
is called the systolic pressure and should be below 140mmHg. With the
end of the ejection of blood by the heart, blood in our arteries runs off
into the distal blood vessels that supply our organs, and the pressure
in the artery will fall. The lowest pressure in the artery, before the next
heartbeat, is the bottom number—90mmHg or below is the normal
range, and is termed the diastolic blood pressure.

HOLTER MONITOR   A device that records an EKG continuously for 24
to 48 hours, then plays back its readings in ultrafast mode through a
computer and allows a doctor to monitor fast, irregular, or unusual
heartbeats. The Holter Monitor, the size of a small portable radio, is
worn on a shoulder strap or clipped to a belt with five wires with small
adhesive electrodes that attach to the chest.

HOMEOPATHY   An alternative medicine system of treatment that is
based on the "principle of similars," the belief that a high dose of a
certain medication produces symptoms similar to specific diseases and
that lower doses of these same medications are effective in treating the
symptoms of the disease.

HOMOCYSTEINE   An amino acid that promotes plaque development in the arteries. High homocysteine levels in the blood are a risk factor for heart disease.

HYPERLIPIDEMIA   Another name for abnormal cholesterol levels in the blood.

INTERCESSORY PRAYER   A form of prayer or meditation in which there is a belief in God who will intercede on our behalf; 96 percent of Americans believe in God, according to a 1996 study published in *JAMA*.

INTRAVASCULAR ULTRASOUND   An angiographic technique that uses a tiny ultrasound crystal at the tip of a wire threaded through the coronary arteries that provides images of specific slices though the artery showing the size of the plaque and the extent to which it is inside the wall. This test gives doctors more information than the angiogram, which can only show how narrow the blood vessel has become. This test, however, involves the same risks as the angiogram and the additional risk of threading a wire through the coronary artery. It is thus not routinely used to detect the existence of plaques.

ISCHEMIA   An insufficient supply of blood to heart muscle, often causing chest pain and often the first indication of heart disease affecting the coronary arteries.

ISOFLAVONES   Found in soy proteins and known to lower cholesterol, these substances are rich in the antioxidants known to have a role in reducing a necessary step in the formation of plaques in our blood vessels.

JAMA   Acronym for the *Journal of the American Medical Association*.

LDL   Low-density lipids, also known as "bad" cholesterol (large and lightweight), the major contributor to the total cholesterol measurement and the most predictive of heart disease risk in populations and patients.

LIPID PROFILE   Three separate groups of particles (LDL cholesterol, HDL cholesterol, and triglycerides) that, along with total cholesterol (the sum of cholesterol in all the lipoprotein particles), are reported as part of any blood test and, if present in abnormal levels, may indicate whether the patient has increased risk of atherosclerosis and consequent heart attacks and strokes.

Lp(a) ("lipoprotein Little A")   A blood particle that may promote plaque growth and clotting. Elevated levels of Lp(a)—over 30 units—are usually inherited and have been shown to increase risk of heart attacks and strokes in some groups of people, especially if LDL cholesterol is also elevated.

lumen   The inside opening of the coronary arteries.

macrophages   White blood cells attracted into the wall of the artery that "gobble up" oxidized LDL cholesterol. When the macrophage is full of oxidized LDL cholesterol, it is called a "foam cell" and is a key component to plaque formation and the process of atherosclerosis in blood vessels.

Mediterranean diet   A diet rich in seafood, fresh fruits, vegetables, and olive oil, and low in saturated (animal) fat, and shown in the Lyon Heart Study to be cardioprotective.

metabolic syndrome   A particularly high-risk combination of obesity, low HDL lipoproteins, high triglycerides, and elevated blood pressure and fasting blood sugar that indicates enhanced risk for developing heart disease.

micronutrients   Small molecules that are not usually sources of energy but play critical roles in the body's function. Micronutrients include vitamins, minerals, flavanoids, and other chemicals.

MRI (also CT) coronary angiography   A diagnostic test using high resolution X-ray and MRI-generated images of the beating heart and the coronary arteries. These images are used to detect and measure obstruction caused by atherosclerotic plaques.

Multiple Risk Factor Intervention Trial (**MRFIT**)   A long-term study of risk factors and heart disease in American men, that confirmed, among other things, the Framingham study's findings that high total cholesterol was associated with a significant increase in heart attack risk over a six-year period.

myopathy   Serious muscle toxicity causing weakness or pain, sometimes an unacceptable side effect of statins when the drugs are taken at maximum dosages.

NIACIN   A B vitamin known, in doses greater than one gram a day, to raise HDL cholesterol and lower triglycerides.

NORMAL SINUS RHYTHM   The electrical impulse that controls the heartbeat; it starts in the upper area of the heart called the sinus node and travels down the heart in an orderly way. An interruption to this orderly process causes a changed pattern of heartbeats called an arrhythmia.

OMEGA-3 OILS   The oils found in fish that are thought to be cardio-protective. *See also* FATS.

PACEMAKER   A small device (about the size of a stack of three half-dollars) used in treating arrhythmias. A pacemaker is placed under the skin with wires threaded through a vein, in the right atrium and ventricle. The pacemaker will sense the electrical activity of the atria and the ventricles, and will stimulate either chamber to "beat" in the case of a blockage or a long pause.

PERCUTANEOUS TRANS CORONARY ANGIOPLASTY (OFTEN REFERRED TO AS PTCA, ANGIOPLASTY, OR INTERVENTIONAL CARDIOLOGY) WITH STENT DEPLOYMENT   An angiographic procedure performed in the cardiac catheterization laboratory used to open arteries clogged with plaque to relieve ischemia and angina symptoms.

PERIPHERAL VASCULAR DISEASE   Atherosclerosis in the arteries that carry blood to the legs.

PLAQUE   Areas of cholesterol, cells, and other proteins that form in the intimal layer of blood vessels and either remain stable and may grow to block the artery and cause ischemia and angina pectoris, or may become unstable and rupture to form the thrombi (blood clots) that cause heart attacks.

PROTEINS   A macronutrient composed of small molecules called amino acids that can be metabolized to produce energy or are used by the body to synthesize most of its critical structural and chemical components. Proteins produce 4 calories per gram. Proteins should make up 15 to 20 percent of a person's daily calories.

RATE OF PERCEIVED EXERTION (RPE)   A method of measuring the intensity of a workout that has as its underlying premise the notion that the mind "knows" how much exercise the body is doing and can identify the optimal 60 to 80 percent of maximum exercise level used in exercise training, thereby eliminating the need to check the pulse or use heart rate monitor during exercise.

REGISTERED DIETICIAN (RD)   A trained and certified nutritionist who helps patients modify their diet and reduce daily calories. The RD is also trained to help a patient develop behavior skills to remain focused and motivated throughout this process.

RESTENOSIS   *See* PERCUTANEOUS TRANS CORONARY ANGIOPLASTY.

RHABDOMYOLISIS   A life-threatening complication and very rare side effect of statin treatment, where muscle cells die rapidly and release into the blood proteins that can cause kidney failure.

ST DEPRESSION (**or ST** SEGMENT DEPRESSION)   A change in an EKG reading indicating that part of the heart is becoming short of blood and oxygen, usually because of a narrowed coronary artery. Another reason that ST segment depression can occur with exercise is certain drugs (such as digitalis) that the patient is taking. Tests on such patients may produce "false positive" results because there is ST depression but no coronary artery disease.

STANOLS   The vegetable version of the cholesterol known to lower LDL cholesterol when part of a diet.

STATINS   A class of drugs that inhibit a critical step in the liver's production of LDL cholesterol. Statins allow physicians to safely reduce LDL cholesterol by up to 50 percent in the overwhelming majority of patients.

SVT (SUPRAVENTICULAR TACHYCARDIA)   A rapid regular heartbeat that usually starts in the atrial chambers at the top of the heart or in the "junction" between the atria and the lower ventricles. It can sometimes be corrected with medications, but is now often "cured" by a proce-dure called electrophysiology with radio frequency ablation. In this procedure, wires are placed in the heart in the same manner as in a car-diac catheterization. The "short circuits" in the conduction pathway responsible for the arrhythmia are identified and destroyed with a small energy pulse.

SYMPATHETIC NERVOUS SYSTEM   Activated during periods of physical and psychological stress and results in an increase in heart rate from impulses that travel down the sympathetic nerves to the heart. In addi-tion, the sympathetic nervous system acts on the adrenal glands (located on the sides of our body right above the kidneys) to produce adrenaline in the bloodstream, which stimulates the heart muscles to contract more forcefully and dilates or constricts blood vessels in var-ious parts of the body. The sympathetic system acts as part of the "fight or flight" response; it is not consciously controlled.

SYSTOLIC PRESSURE   *See* HIGH BLOOD PRESSURE.

THALLIUM STRESS TEST   *See* EXERCISE STRESS NUCLEAR IMAGING.

TRIGLYCERIDES   Particles made up of small sugarlike molecules called glycerol and three attached fatty acid molecules; which, when elevated in the blood, are predictors or indicators of heart disease. High triglyc-erides are part of the metabolic syndrome in patients who have central obesity and other risk factors.

TSH (THYROID STIMULATING HORMONE)   This is a blood test of thy-roid function. An underactive thyroid gland, called hypothyroidism, will often be associated with high cholesterol values and treatment of the thyroid disorder may result in these values returning to normal.

TYPE A BEHAVIOR   First noted by Dr. Friedman and Rosenman, a per-sonality type distinguished by three characteristics: time urgency, com-petitiveness, and free-floating hostility. Known to be a risk factor for heart disease.

TYPE D PERSONALITY   A combination of "distress" emotions that includes anger, anxiety, and depression. If present in a person's emotional makeup, this behavior pattern signifies coronary heart disease risk.

UNSTABLE CORONARY SYNDROME   Symptoms of angina pectoris (chest pain) that are increasing, coming on at rest, or associated with important changes on the patient's electrocardiogram and elevations of the cardiac blood markers that indicate damage to heart muscle cells. Such conditions are often a good reason to do an immediate coronary angiogram.

"VAGAL" NERVOUS SYSTEM   Named after the major nerve in this system and another name for the parasympathetic nervous system. Impulses from this system slow the heart, lower blood pressure, and increase the digestion.

VENTRICULAR FIBRILLATION   The loss of organized electrical activity in the heart that is always associated with loss of effective heartbeats. This electrical activity is the wavy line seen on the monitors in the ER TV shows and will lead to death unless it is shocked (defibrillated) back to normal.

VPCs   (VENTRICULAR PREMATURE CONTRACTIONS) This is a kind of arrhythmia. *See* APCs.

Appendix I

BODY MASS INDEX (BMI) CHART

The following chart converts pounds and inches to a BMI number (usually figured in kilograms and meters). You have a healthy BMI if your score is up to 24.9, you are overweight if your score is 25 to 29.9, and you are obese if your score is over 29.9.

BMI (KG/M2)	19	20	21	22	23	24	25	26	27	28	29	30	35	40
Height (in.)	Weight (lb.)													
58	91	96	100	105	110	115	119	124	129	134	138	143	167	191
59	94	99	104	109	114	119	124	128	133	138	143	148	173	198
60	97	102	107	112	118	123	128	133	138	143	148	153	179	204
61	100	106	111	116	122	127	132	137	143	148	153	158	185	211
62	104	109	115	120	126	131	136	142	147	153	158	164	191	218
63	107	113	118	124	130	135	141	146	152	158	163	169	197	225
64	110	116	122	128	134	140	145	151	157	163	169	174	204	232
65	114	120	126	132	138	144	150	156	162	168	174	180	210	240
66	118	124	130	136	142	148	155	161	167	173	179	186	216	247
67	121	127	134	140	146	153	159	166	172	178	185	191	223	255
68	125	131	138	144	151	158	164	171	177	184	190	197	230	262
69	128	135	142	149	155	162	169	176	182	189	196	203	236	270
70	132	139	146	153	160	167	174	181	188	195	202	207	243	278
71	136	143	150	157	165	172	179	186	193	200	208	215	250	286
72	140	147	154	162	169	177	184	191	199	206	213	221	258	294
73	144	151	159	166	174	182	189	197	204	212	219	227	265	302
74	148	155	163	171	179	186	194	202	210	218	225	233	272	311
75	152	160	168	176	184	192	200	208	216	224	232	240	279	319
76	156	164	172	180	189	197	205	213	221	230	238	246	287	328

Body mass index according to height in inches and weight in pounds.

Appendix II

RISK OF ASSOCIATED DISEASE ACCORDING TO BMI AND WAIST SIZE

The chart below estimates a person's overall risk of disease if he or she is overweight or obese. At each BMI level (on the left of the chart), the risk is higher if waist size measures more than 35 inches in a woman or 40 inches in a man (two right columns on the chart).

RISK OF ASSOCIATED DISEASE ACCORDING TO BMI AND WAIST SIZE			
BMI		Waist less than or equal to 40 in. (men) or 35 in. (women)	Waist greater than 40 in. (men) or 35 in. (women)
18.5 or less	Underweight	——	N/A
18.5–24.9	Normal	——	N/A
25.0–29.9	Overweight	Increased	High
30.0–34.9	Obese	High	Very High
35.0–39.9	Very Obese	High	Very High
40 or greater	Extremely Obese	Extremely High	Extremely High

Appendix III

REVISED RATED PERCEIVED EXERTION SCALE (1–10) DEVELOPED BY DR. GUNNAR BORG

0	Nothing at all
0.5	Very, very weak
1	Very weak
2	Weak
3	Moderate
4	Somewhat strong
5	Strong
6	
7	Very strong
8	
9	
10	Very, very strong

As you are exercising, describe how intense your exertion feels, using the words on the 1–10 scale.

Appendix IV

WEBSITES FOR HELPFUL INFORMATION ABOUT NEW RULES TOPICS

1. General

www.americanheart.org The American Heart Association's website. It is a source of excellent information on all aspects of heart disease and risk as they relate to the New Rules.

2. Diet

www.nal.uda.gov/fnic The U.S. Department of Agriculture's library website. It is a very good source of diet information, with links to other good sites.

www.eatright.org The American Dietetic Association's website. It contains excellent information and helpful practical tips.

3. Exercise

www.acsm.org The website of the American College of Sports and Medicine. Excellent exercise and fitness information.

www.chosefitness.com A good site for information about starting an exercise program.

www.health.msn.com Very good articles on many aspects of health, including exercise.

4. Smoking Cessation

www.nlm.nih.gov/medicineplus/smokingcessation The website of the National Institutes of Health devoted to information about the dangers of smoking. It also offers successful programs to stop smoking.

www.ahrq.gov/consumer/tobacco Excellent information on starting a smoking cessation program.

www.surgeongeneral.gov/tobacco/consquits Offers excellent information and is a good way to start your own smoking cessation program.

5. Cholesterol and Lipids

www.nhlbi.nih.gov/chd The website for the National Cholesterol Education Program. Excellent information.

www.nhlbisupport.com/chd1/meds The National Heart, Lung, and Blood Institute (NHLBI) of the National Institutes of Health. The website is a consumer-friendly site that addresses the use of medications to lower cholesterol.

www.hsph.harvard.edu/nutritionsource/fats A good source of information about diet changes to lower cholesterol.

6. Alternative and Complementary Medicine

www.nccam.nih.gov National Center of Complementary and Alternative Medicine. Excellent balanced information.

www.herbmed.org Evidenced-based information on supplements and herbs.

Complementary and Alternative Cardiovascular Medicine A textbook coedited by Dr. Richard Stein and Dr. Mehmet Oz (Humana Press Inc., 1999). Dr. Oz and I produced this book for physicians, but most of the information is accessible to the general public.

Acknowledgments

My friends and colleagues at SUNY Downstate are all, in important ways, responsible for the thinking behind this book: Dr. Norman Krasnow, my chief of cardiology, who helped me to grow as a doctor and a teacher; Florence Frank, RN, who started the cardiac exercise lab with me; and my friend Roseann Chesler, EdD, who continues to share my excitement and curiosity about what exercise does and how it does it.

The American Heart Association in New York and in the national offices are comprised of a unique and dedicated group of professionals and volunteers who have made my career much more interesting and rewarding than it would have been otherwise. Michael Weamer, the executive vice president of the Heritage Affiliate (encompassing New York, New Jersey, and Connecticut), Alice Austin, Fred Gomez, Susan Bishop, Darcy Spitz, and Julie Delbarto are among my friends at "Heart." Their dedication and talent have continually challenged me to grow and to think. Risk Platt, RD, is a good friend, wonderful nutritionist, and fellow volunteer at the American Heart Association. I call upon her knowledge and experience often.

The 92nd Street Y in New York City has been a second professional home for me since 1975 when Dan Kaplan, Chuck Bronz, Dr. Arthur Aufsus, and I started the Cardiac Prevention and Rehabilitation Program. This organization continues to provide an extraordinary program to New Yorkers with heart disease, due in large part to the wonderful people at the Y, many of whom are treasured friends: Sol Adler, Miribai Holland (who encouraged me to write about the New Rules), Dave Schmeltzer, Barbara Bentley, my longtime friend Herb Saltzman, and my friend and colleague Dr. Nieca Goldberg, who serves with me as director of the Cardiac Program at the Y and has played an important role in changing how women and their doctors think about heart disease.

Esther Margolis, president and publisher of Newmarket Press, and senior editor Keith Hollaman shared my passion about the New Rules for outliving heart disease and were essential sources of guidance in turning that passion into a book. Susan A. Schwartz worked closely with me as an editor and writer to produce a completed manuscript, and much of what I like best about the book reflects her skills.

Index

About the Author

Dr. Richard A. Stein is a Professor of Medicine and Director of the Urban Community Cardiology Program at New York University School of Medicine. His former positions include Director of Preventive Cardiology at Beth Israel Medical Center; Director of the Beth Israel–Long Island College Hospital Cardiology Fellowship Program; Chief of Medicine at the Singer Hospital of Beth Israel Hospital in New York; and Professor of Medicine and Chief of Cardiology at the State University of New York–Downstate Medical Center in Brooklyn. He is the founder and co-director of the Cardiac Exercise and Intervention Program at the 92nd Street Y in New York City. A long-standing National Media Spokesperson for the American Heart Association, he currently serves as Co-President of the AHA's Founders Affiliate, comprising New York, New Jersey, Connecticut, Massachusetts, Vermont, Rhode Island, New Hampshire, and Maine. Dr. Stein has published over 65 articles and chapters in professional publications, and is a recipient of the U.S. National Institutes of Health's Preventive Cardiology Academic Award. He is co-editor, along with Dr. Mehmet Oz, of a textbook for physicians on complementary and alternative cardiovascular medicine. Dr. Stein divides his time between New York City and Connecticut.